FIT MOM SECRETS

How to Get Into Shape and Stay
in Shape with Children at Home

CHRISTINA L. MORELAND

DEDICATIONS

To my sons, Ashton and Luke:

Thank you for the daily inspiration and for the many adventures! I love you both more than you can possibly imagine.

And to my husband, Lance:

Thank you for believing in me and for the constant support and encouragement.

Legal Disclaimers & Copyright Info

CONTENTS

I INVITE YOU...

Welcome to *Fit Mom Secrets*! Before we get started, I wanted to let you know about an interactive program I offer, called the Super Mom Get Fit program, to help moms get back into shape working more closely with me. The information you're about to read in this book has the ability to change your life for the better, but it's only as good as your ability to stay motivated and apply the lessons within.

But my Super Mom Get Fit program is fully interactive and walks you through step by step on what to do, when, and takes the guesswork — and the intimidation factor — out of going to the gym. If you'd like to work with me more closely, I invite you to consider the Super Mom Get Fit program, where you'll get immediate access to everything inside the membership program, including:

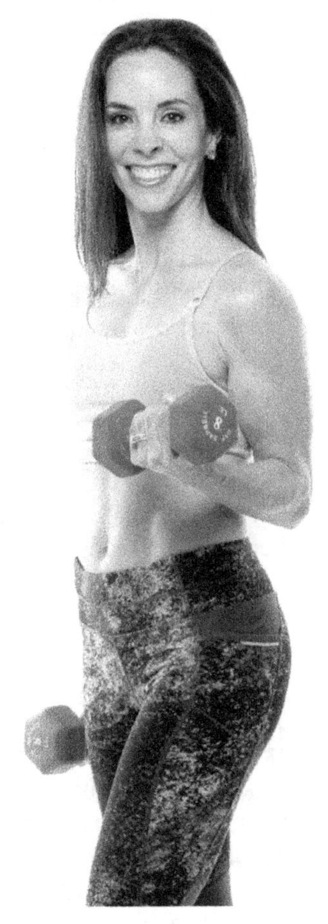

- ✓ the video workouts demonstrating how I shed that 12% body fat in just 4 months

- ✓ 12-week Advanced workout for moms with kids of all ages

- ✓ 6 weeks of postpartum exercises you can do with your baby at home

- ✓ access to a private support community on Facebook

- ✓ weekly motivation

- ✓ printable success journals, nutrition log, and more...

And the Super Mom Get Fit program is for **all** moms who want to get into a sustainable healthy lifestyle, even if you have kids at home. You'll never have to go into the gym and wonder what to do again – it's all planned out for you, hitting all muscle groups on a consistent basis, so you get strength and endurance training for a symmetrical, well-balanced, "Fit Mom" body.

Check it out at this link: *www.FitMomSecrets.com/Book-Offer*

INTRODUCTION

Before I Had Kids...

You'll start so many sentences that way from now on. But before I had children, my husband, Lance, and I were visiting some family at his aunt's house over a summer weekend. His mother and aunt were being complimentary when they said I looked thin that day — women will often use the words "thin" or "skinny" when they really mean "fit and lean." I thanked them for the compliment, but right after that someone else in the room said, *"Just wait until she has kids."*

I was struck and just stood there, stunned. *Is it possible that this is the time in my life when I'm at my most fit and vibrant?* I wondered. Suddenly I began mourning the potential loss of something I still had — my fitness — because I wasn't yet able to experience whether it was possible or impossible to get my body back after having babies. And even if I could do it after the first child, what about the second, or the third, and so on?

Have you wondered the same thing? Or have you never even considered the possibility that you could have an even *better,* fitter body after having children, because you thought that's just something we inevitably sacrifice to Motherhood? I hope to change your mind with this book! Because not only is it possible to get back in shape, it's possible to get into even *better* shape than before you got pregnant. Now that's something to get really excited about!

Is This All There Is?

Aside from forfeiting our physical identity when we have a baby, even if it's just temporarily, many of us experience a surprising and distressing identity crisis on a deeply personal level when we confront the changing roles of our Mom identity head-on. We literally go from being an individual to a parent overnight, and the reality of those changes, even though we thought we knew what to expect, is sometimes difficult to accept — even when you're madly in love with your new precious baby or thriving with your older children.

And I understand because I've been there. Some days you wonder, even if just to yourself, *is there anything more? What am I doing here? What's my purpose?* Your primary and most essential purpose as a mother is obvious, of course — it's to care for and love your children. But what about beyond that?

Having children might complete you in one area of your life, but we're human beings. We are complex, and our social needs are many – professional, spiritual, marital — it's normal to want some things for your life outside of your children.

And it's an important question to answer for yourself, because sometimes the answers don't come for a long time. Asking these questions is one of the main reasons why I wrote this book and why I feel so strongly about reclaiming your physical fitness and identity after children.

Why do I think this is important? *Because this is you defining your new identity and maintaining a sense of who you were, and are, outside of your role as Mom.* Despite all my experiences as a mother over the past 10 years, I'm still Christina. And it's important for me to know that and to like who I am — I mean, we have to spend all day long with ourselves, you might as well know and love that person!

Reclaiming your physical fitness is the air beneath your wings to allow you to soar and give back in the best possible way… You become stronger, and therefore, more confident. You become happier, and that joy radiates to others. You become refreshed, and therefore, able to give back to your family with more enthusiasm and grace. Essentially, getting back into amazing shape allows you to be an even better giver than you already are — to your family, friends, and everyone else you encounter. **You become a blessing.** And it creates a Ripple Effect on the rest of your life.

This One's for You!

Fit Mom Secrets is all for YOU, and I won't let you become the forgotten woman! That's why in this book I'll help you remember the individual inside you, who is still there and needs to be recognized, even when you're juggling children, a job, and a full family life.

Putting It All Together

In the section, *"Getting Back Into Super Shape,"* I share my Fit Mom Secrets for how I lost all the baby weight after child number two in just sixteen weeks. Yes, you read that right. Just 4 months and I was back in shape. No gimmicks here; just sound nutrition and exercise. I did it… and you can, too. After all, you're a Super Mom, just like me. And now you can be a Fit Mom, too, for LIFE.

If you've tried other programs in the past and failed, or the program failed you, don't worry about it. If you're a "non-gym-goer" because you get intimidated in a weight room, don't worry about it… I'm offering you an incredible opportunity to check all your past failures and negative experiences out the door. Because this is for you and it's something you can totally do.

What I'm going to share with you will help you get into the best shape of your life!

I want to share this information with you and help you learn what I've learned from working in a sports nutrition company for years, as a certified personal trainer, and from working directly with a clinical nutritionist with more than 30 years of experience to help me with my personal goals…

First, you are never too old or too out of shape to get started…

And second, you CAN change your body. You can even change the shape of your body, with the right information. I'm offering you an amazing opportunity to look and feel better, to be healthier, to be an amazing example to your children and show them you CAN do anything!

To teach them the value of respecting the human form and our amazing ability to accomplish anything we set our minds to. You do the same!

First, I'm going to walk you through a 6-week Postpartum Program that will activate your muscles and allow you to exercise with your baby, if you still have a baby at home. If you're past the 3-month postpartum mark or your kids are older, then great! We'll jump right into the 12-week program that I used to lose 12% body fat in just 4 months.

With this program, I went from 26.8% body fat to just 14.2%, and just a couple of months beyond that 4-month period, I hit an all-time personal fitness record.

So, this plan works!

When you encounter tough days — and believe me — there will be tough days, I want you to think of the PRIZE. Because what you're after HAS to be more desirable than staying in the same place you're in now. Your clothes will start to feel baggy… you'll have more energy… you'll start to see muscle definition where you've never had it before…

And after realizing you can change your body with intention and precision, you will tap into an extraordinary superpower and begin to apply this kind of success to other areas of your life.

So put aside your doubts, your fears, and your excuses. And instead think about the **possibilities.** And let's get to work.

Remember, I'm a mom first, just like you! I'm not a fitness model. I have a unique understanding of your challenges and struggles… I've been there… and I'm still in the trenches of Motherhood with you…

So let's do this!

I'm so excited you're here!!!

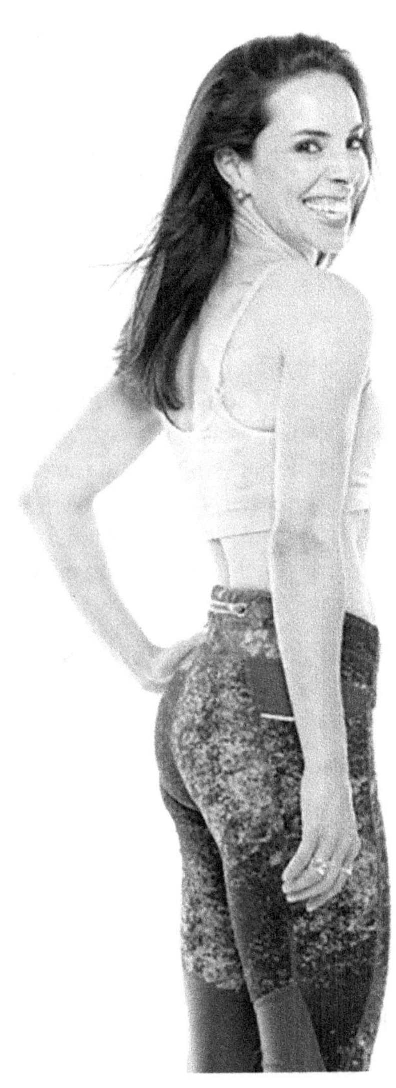

SECTION ONE
SUPER NUTRITION

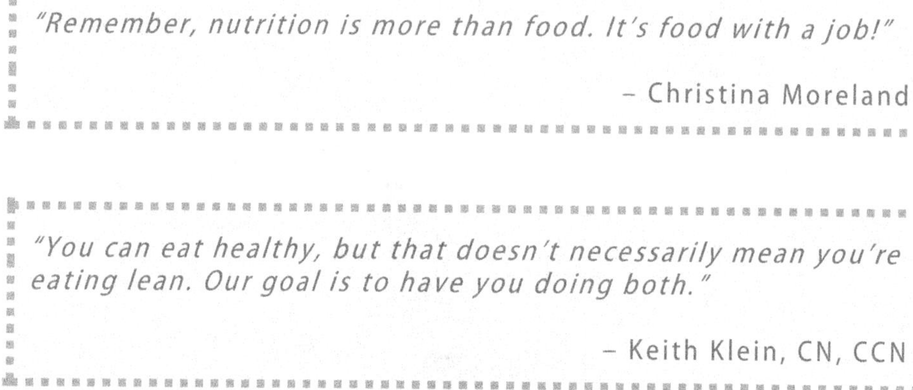

> *"Remember, nutrition is more than food. It's food with a job!"*
>
> – Christina Moreland

> *"You can eat healthy, but that doesn't necessarily mean you're eating lean. Our goal is to have you doing both."*
>
> – Keith Klein, CN, CCN

In the Introduction we talked a lot about how your changing role as a mother can significantly impact your psyche and self-worth. One challenge I was having immediately after Ashton, my oldest, was born, was that I was going through so many enormous changes in my life at the same time. But the other part of maintaining your "Super Self" is the ability to quickly get your body back into shape after having a baby. And like I mentioned in the Introduction, you may not believe this is possible, but I want you to know that you have the Super Power within yourself to create whatever you want for your own life.

I'm not saying that getting your body back will be easy, but it's possible. And it's even possible to not only shed baby weight, or whatever weight you have to lose, within a few short months, but it's also possible to have an even *better* body and physique afterwards.

I always considered myself to be a somewhat serious athlete/runner. In high school, I ran the hundred-meter and two-hundred-meter dashes and did those races on a relay team, often running the first or fourth leg of the race. I was little, but fast! In college, I signed up for running classes because I knew they would keep me in shape, and physical education was required, so I figured I would do something I enjoyed that would help me burn lots of calories.

Back then I didn't know anything about nutrition, other than my ideas of "eating healthy," which involved buying anything that said "reduced fat" or "fat free."

I avoided indulging in pizza and beer late at night like my friends; I kept my portions small, and tried to avoid greasy, fried foods. I knew nothing about power foods (foods that increase your body's performance) or body fat percentages, I didn't know that you could weigh less on the scale but still be fatter than before (what my nutritionist calls "skinny fat"), or that skipping meals makes you store more fat, or that resistance training is the only way to change body *shape*.

FIT MOM SECRET:

Running is a great form of physical exercise and is good for your heart, but the only way to change body *shape* is to use resistance training with weights.

Intense cardio, such as running or cycling, will make you a smaller version of yourself, but if you want to change body shape, resistance is the way to go.

Fast-forward fifteen years – I've had a career, home and family life and two children. I still enjoy running, but the difference for me is that it's now about enjoying the run, the journey of being outdoors, not the end result of increased speed or stamina – although it's still fun to do sprints and it happens to also be a great exercise for the quadriceps and glutes. Why has my attitude toward it changed? Because of what I have learned within that timeframe, mainly from working in the fitness industry for the past several years.

Here in *Fit Mom Secrets*, I'm going to share it all with you – some things you may have heard or read, some you haven't. I'll give you my insider tips of how to plan healthy meals for the family while you work to reach your own fitness goals. Because now that you're a mom, you've also become a consummate juggler of time. You need to be able to maximize your time in the gym or at home while exercising, and still get amazing results.

See, one thing that happened while I was in college significantly impacted how I viewed nutrition and physical fitness: *as a means to an end,* simply a way to get me where I wanted to go. Like I've said, I always enjoyed it and cared about being fit, but while I was a sophomore in college my mother began competing in amateur bodybuilding competitions. Yep, you read that correctly. My mother, who was in her late forties at the time, *started* working out for the first time in her life while I was studying at Texas A&M University.

And I didn't realize it at the time, but observing my mom's fitness journey while I was nineteen and surrounded with tempting unhealthy choices, significantly changed my life.

She and a few girlfriends had made a pact: they would get into the best shape of their lives, and they would do it together, supporting one another the entire way. As a motivator, they each signed up for an upcoming figure bodybuilding show and then worked like crazy to reach their goals. At first I thought my mother was insane. *"You're going to do WHAT?!?"* It's possible the word "CRAZY" even came out of my mouth. But once I was there I realized something really important.

In order to reach a goal of any kind, you have to set mini goals along the way to propel you forward.

Mom's upcoming competition was just a date in her calendar that she would work toward, and obviously the thought of being on a huge stage in front of hundreds of people wearing nothing but a skimpy bikini will certainly motivate you to perform!

Life is funny, and I don't believe in chance. Through my mother's lifestyle change I met two people who have forever changed my life and the way I think about taking care of my body, Lee Labrada and nutritionist Keith Klein. Their involvement in my life has also impacted how I teach my children about making good food choices and incorporating exercise as a part of daily life.

Nutrition Guru

To prepare for her show, Mom worked with renown nutritionist Keith Klein, CN, CCN, for weeks. He taught her how to calculate the fat percentages in foods and which foods to avoid, how to make sure you're consuming enough calories to support any dietary or fitness goal, and how to train muscles properly to get them to respond. When I met him at nineteen, I had no interest in competing, but benefited significantly from what I saw my mother doing.

Backstage at Mom's show I saw how all the competitors prepared for their few minutes on stage. Up until that point they had all been training for the past twelve – sixteen weeks or longer, which included daily workouts and preparing and consuming between five and six lean balanced meals a day.

As the competitors awaited to be called on stage they drank from their gallon jugs of water, snacked on mini meals they had packed into coolers, wore robes to prevent the suntan spray from streaking, had spray tan on-hand for touchups, music for their routines, an extra pair of clothes, along with an extra swimsuit. **In other words, they were prepared and dedicated athletes who had worked up to this single moment for weeks.**

On stage, my mom rocked it! Cheers erupted from the crowd and she took home a third-place trophy on top of that! **I couldn't have been more proud, but at the same time I realized that she couldn't have possibly done all of that without the right tools, motivation and knowledge.**

Although I initially met Keith Klein when I was nineteen and had no interest in figure competition, our meeting was serendipitous, and he's changed my life with his vast knowledge, support, encouragement and friendship.

In addition to teaching you how to drop unwanted body fat and increase *your* metabolism, the important lean and clean principles I've learned for my own body translate to how I plan meals, cook and serve my husband and boys. It's not just your health that's at stake here, after all, it's also your children's. I hope to teach you some principles you can use for the rest of your life and set in motion a lasting positive difference for you that will help you to create and sustain a healthy *family*.

Learning how to plan meals early on for you and your baby sets the tone for a healthy child later. After reading this chapter, you will know what to eat and how to shop for whole nutritious foods, have a sample meal plan to make it easier for you to create delicious healthy foods for yourself and family, and have learned the fundamentals of how to lose your baby weight and get into the best shape of your life.

I'll give you the right tools (information), but the determination and consistency have to come from you. I'll tell you what has worked for me and for others who have been successful, but succeeding in this area does require commitment and follow-through. I know you can do it!

Meal Planning 101

Now, what if I could give you some family-tested lean and healthy recipes that are easy to make on the fly or prepare early in the week so you reach your goal of feeding your family nutritious and delicious foods? There are several keys to success here.

- Lean and healthy food can, and should be delicious.

- Early preparation and planning are critical to achieving meals that contain the balance of protein, carbohydrates and fats you'll need to feed yourself and your kids.

- We need color and variety in foods to achieve satiety.

➡ You'll be more successful with this program, and in the long run, if you can change your mentality to first consider what *nutritional benefit* the food you're serving offers, THEN think about how to make it delicious.

One thing that's very different about what I'll present in this chapter versus what you may have read in outside sources about diet and nutrition, is that I'm combining your meal plan and your child's. The reason I'm presenting it that way is because as a mother I know how incredibly difficult it can be to get everyone the basic foods they need to function throughout the day, and to do it on time! You shouldn't have to worry about preparing something completely different from what your children eat because you have weight loss and fitness goals. **You won't eat the same proportions of foods as your baby or toddler, obviously, and babies need additional fat in some cases, but for the most part, you and your family can and should eat the same meals after your baby is twelve months or older.**

I'll point out where you can easily modify for your baby's growing needs. I'll show you how to be strategic and maximize your time in the kitchen and at mealtimes. The winning result will be that your baby gets wonderful healthy meals and you progressively build muscle, burn fat, speed up your metabolism and end up with the body of your dreams. Are you excited yet?

In order to eat healthy you need to know:

➡ **What to eat**

➡ **When to eat it**

➡ **How much of it to eat**

That's it!

Now I'm going to borrow an illustration from my good friend, Lee Labrada. Lee is THE master when it comes to building muscle, burning fat and understanding nutrition. He is a former professional bodybuilder, best selling author of *The Lean Body Promise,* and president and CEO of Labrada Nutrition, maker of wonderful sports nutrition supplements for athletes, fitness enthusiasts, and the average person trying to get into better shape.

Lee says when serving yourself food proportions, you should first divide your plate into thirds:

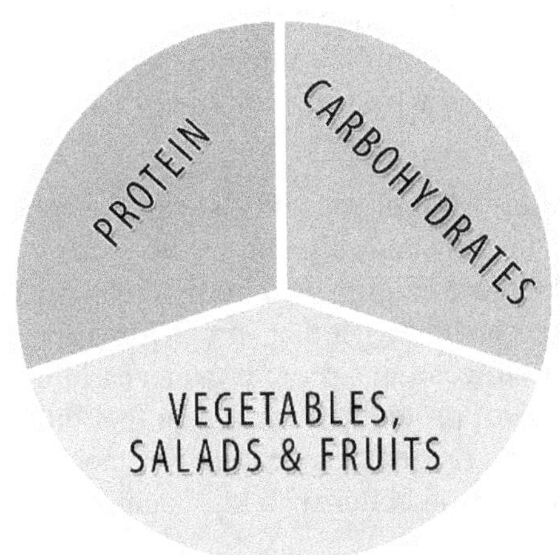

The Rule of Thirds

Imagine your full-sized dinner plate in front of you and then visually split it into equal thirds. Cover one third of your plate with a protein source, the next third with a complex carbohydrate, and the final third with a vegetable, salad or fruit. I'll show you examples in just a minute.

When serving a meal to a baby on solid foods or a toddler, you can do the same thing on a smaller plate meant for his age group.

The first third, made up of the protein, is the single most important portion of your meal. Make sure to always incorporate a protein into every meal, no matter what. The reason why the protein is so important is that protein fuels your muscle, and the more muscle you have, the more fat you will burn, even at rest. That's right, you heard me correctly!

The more muscle you have, the more fat and calories you'll burn, even just sitting at your desk or riding in a car.

Building muscle and strength also helps to support other important bodily tissue, such as your joints and cartilage. And your muscles support good bone health. Often, rheumatologists and orthopedic specialists tell their patients to do strength-training exercises to prevent muscle atrophy (muscle loss) as a result of the muscles not being worked enough. So, building muscle is a good thing, ladies. The heavier you can lift over time, the more you'll put nice definition in the right places.

And trust me, you WON'T LOOK LIKE MEN! But more on that later when we get to the workout chapter. For now, I simply wanted to explain why protein is so important for you and for your family, and why you want to start with your protein at every meal.

So the first reason you want to begin your meals with a protein is because protein is what keeps your muscles healthy and full, and we've already talked about how the more muscle you have the more calories you burn at rest. Secondly, protein takes longer for the body to absorb and digest than simple or complex carbohydrates, so you actually burn more calories digesting a protein than a carbohydrate. Thirdly, when you consume adequate amounts of protein per meal, you feel fuller longer and are more satiated, thereby reducing the risk of binge eating or snacking on the wrong foods. And lastly, major organs function better with high quality protein.

Consuming protein provides your body with essential amino acids, used to communicate properly with the brain, and protein plays a crucial part in brain development and function, which is why it's so important for your child. Neurotransmitters are the brain's communication channels, and they help to maintain proper natural levels of chemicals such as serotonin, epinephrine and dopamine, which regulate moods and assist with concentration, memory and learning ability.

Most neurotransmitters are made from amino acids acquired from the protein in the foods you consume. They are the brain chemicals that help you do everything, including focus, concentrate or feel relaxed. They can excite or calm your brain and can shift your mood or change your mind. What you eat affects which nerve chemicals will be dominant in your brain, and this can affect how you feel. That's why it's essential to get good quality foods at regular intervals throughout the day.

Quick and Easy Measuring

A quick and simple way to "measure" out your food just by eyeballing it is to use your palm and fist. Your palm is roughly the size of a 4 – 5 ounce chicken breast. And your fist is the size of the complex carbohydrate and vegetables, roughly 3/4 cup - 1 cup. We covered basic nutrition for babies in *Secrets of the Super Moms, Part I,* but when your baby becomes a toddler, you can do the same thing as you do with your own meals: start with the protein source, but use smaller portions.

Our pediatrician always told us that babies are generally good self-regulating eaters when it comes to portions – they will stop when they're full. Ironically, even though toddlers are more active than infants, their caloric requirements decrease. But good nutrition is still important and cutting total calories does not mean you should shortcut any of the essentials – proteins, complex carbohydrates, vegetables, fruits and essential fats – for them either.

Start every meal with a protein base because that's the brain food, and then make sure to add in a complex carbohydrate and vegetable, and the protein and balanced nutrients will help to satiate you until the next meal. So remember, hand and fist. It's easy!

What a Fit Mom Eats

Now that you know how to measure your food, let's talk about what to eat. Most fitness experts and fat loss gurus tell you what to avoid. Well, duh! Most of us know what we *can't* have, but we need to know what we *can* and *should* have to boost our metabolisms, build strong healthy kids, and maximize our fat loss goals. So, I'm going to give you the basics and then we'll break it down.

To begin eating lean, first we have to reset your mind to think in terms of eating five small meals every day, rather than three. And in many cases, you're so busy as a mom that you may even be skipping meals. Stop that right now! You must eat frequently to kick-start your metabolism and rev it up to burn unwanted body fat. This is because when you skip meals your body actually goes into a "panic" mode and instead of slowly digesting the food over time, it stores it up. So when you skip meals you're actually teaching your body to take whatever next meal you eat and **turn it into fat**.

Understanding Food Labels

Secondly, eating lean is about keeping the total fat in meals to under 20 percent fat calories. This can be very difficult to do, as most food products have confusing and misleading labeling. (It's actually a trick food manufacturers bank on you falling for when you're trying to buy "healthy" foods. "Healthy" does not necessarily also mean "lean," and what you really want is *lean* foods if you have a dietary or fitness goal that requires you to shed some body fat or increase your metabolism, or both.)

But don't worry, I'll show you how to calculate accurately what you're eating every single time. Once you have this basic formula down, you don't need a calculator any more, but at first, I'd like to suggest you bring one with you to the supermarket when you go shopping. It will help big time, trust me!

Thirdly, there is another popular term that's been widely publicized recently and causing a lot of confusion, and it's called *eating clean*. While eating *lean* is about keeping foods to a certain fat percentage, *eating clean* is about eating foods in their most natural form. For lean meats, that means without a lot of additives or sauces – but it does *not* mean boring or tasteless. For fruits and vegetables, it means consuming them in the form of whole foods, not smothered with cheeses and butter, or adulterated with hormones or chemicals.

Eating clean means avoiding too many processed foods or foods with a ton of added sugar, high levels of saturated and trans fats or foods that have been stripped of their nutritional value by having a lot of hormones or preservatives added to them.

The Real World

Now that we've discussed the difference between *lean* and *clean eating*, I wanted to share a little more background with you. While it's true I never had an interest in competing in figure or bodybuilding competitions like my mother, I was still fascinated by how she had changed her body in just a few short weeks. And she did it at a time in her life when many people would have given up or thought they were too old to begin – she was 48.

It was obvious the training and conditioning helped to build those nice beautiful curves and toned muscles, but the nutrition during that timeframe is what gave her the greatest results possible. I took note, and while I didn't do what she did to a T, I was still able to avoid detrimental temptations at what could have been a time of huge pitfalls for me, while I was attending college.

Let's face it – in college, you're in charge of your destiny for the first time in your life. The people you meet, your class arrangements, when and what you eat, if you drink, when (and if) you do homework, are all within your control and on your own timetable. The "Freshman Fifteen" is an understatement – I had seen some of my friends gain twenty or more pounds within just two months of having all that freedom, and I was determined it would not happen to me.

Still, I didn't yet know the depth of importance of *what* to eat, *when*, and *why*.

After graduation, eating lean became more difficult as I hung out with the work crowd, got invited to happy hours, and became more social as a professional. I knew to avoid most restaurant food and how to cook some basic meals at home to take care of myself. But I wanted to reach my full potential, so I decided to go and see my mom's nutritionist, Keith Klein. I went to him for a personal consultation for the first time when I was twenty-two.

And even though I was doing pretty well with my own plan, my body fat was still at 18 percent, which I thought was high considering my age and genetics. Keith helped me devise meals that fit into my everyday life, that were lean, healthy and helped me reach my fitness goals – which at the time were to maintain a healthy lean body fat percentage, and a toned and fit athletic look.

Within a few weeks and with minimal adjustments, I dropped to 14 percent. I had simply made a few dietary changes – eating more frequently during the day and increasing my protein – and this altered my body chemistry dramatically, although I didn't feel like I had sacrificed a thing.

My personal goals have evolved based on what was happening in my life at the time – whether or not I was pregnant or trying to get pregnant, losing the post-baby fat, or amping up my training to look like a fitness competitor. Keith was my immediate go-to person through all of my pregnancies (I had two miscarriages in between my two boys), and again after I had the second baby and found the recovery much more difficult than it had been the first time. Then again, that wasn't really surprising – at that point not only had I delivered two babies via c-section delivery, which required a surgeon cutting through my entire abdominal muscle wall both times, but I'd also had two miscarriages in between the births of my sons.

My body had to recover from those experiences and the weight fluctuations that were part of each one. Needless to say, I've learned a lot about my own body and about nutrition and fitness over the nineteen years I've been studying the subject – a learning curve that was especially accelerated in the four-year period during which I had my children.

Keith helped me tweak what I was eating and I shed 12 percent body fat within just sixteen weeks after I had Luke.

BODY COMPOSITION

8.5 wks pregnant

MEASURE	DATE	DATE	DATE	DATE	DATE	DATE
	6.21.07	[illegible]	3.5.09	12.8.09	7.26.11	8.16.11
BICEP	8	4	6	9	12	9
ICEP	3	2.5	2	3	6	2
SUBSCAP.	7	8.5	8	9	6	9
SUPRA.	11 (31)	6 (23)	10	14	13	10
IG	2	6	6	6	8	6
ABDOMINAL	7	2	7	9	14	8
KIDNEY	14	16	8.5	5	20	13
IUAD	21.5	16	13	15	22	17
CALVE	6	5	5	4	6	5
TOTAL	80.5	[illegible]	63.5	70	107	83
BODYWEIGHT						
	79	113	64	66	93	71
%FAT	18%	[illegible]	14.1%	18.1% / 24.5	26.4%	30.85%
FAT POUNDS	15.10	12.52	13.45	15.42	22.64	23.40
LEAN BODYMASS	[illegible]	[illegible]	85.04	36.51	74.85	85.07

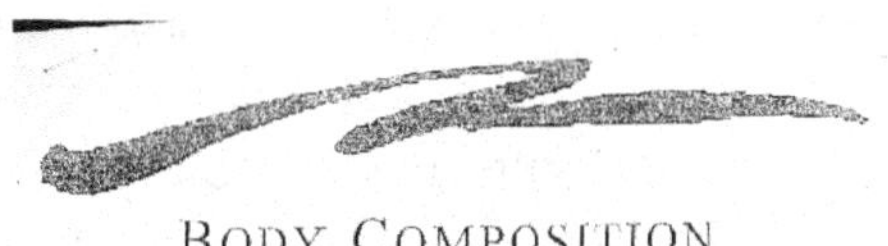

BODY COMPOSITION

MEASURE	DATE	DATE	DATE	DATE	DATE	DATE
	9.8.11	10.4.11	11.15.11	3.25.12		
TRICEP	6	7	7	5		
BICEP	2	1.5	2	1		
SUBSCAP.	8	8	7	6		
SUPRA.	9	8	7	5		
ITC	4	4	3	2		
ABDOMINAL	7	8	7	5		
KIDNEY	13	10	7	7		
QUAD	15	18	14	9		
CALVE	3	3	3	2		
TOTAL	70	63.5	55	42		
BODYWEIGHT						
	46	60	53	43		
%FAT	17.3%	16.2%	14.31%	11.6%		
FAT POUNDS	14.16	12.01	14.75	11.14		
LEAN BODYMASS	87.13	87.73	88.44	85.30		

If you take a look at my body fat measurements shown here, I want to point out a few simple things. First, I started at 26.4 percent body fat, or 28.64 fat pounds. The number of fat pounds means how many total pounds of fat you have in your body at that particular time. Your body must have some fat to support itself, vital organs and regular basic function. So having some fat is not a bad thing, but my goal post-baby was to get to an athletic body fat for my size, height and activity level, which for me is under 14 percent.

It could be 17 percent for you – it just depends on how you look, feel and function – so let these numbers be a guide, but don't feel you should try to match them, because your body chemistry is different from mine.

The Scale is a Big FAT Lie!

After Keith and I changed my nutrition plan, I was at 14.3 percent body fat by November, just four months later, and only had 14.73 total fat pounds. My total body fat had dropped 12.1 percent in only sixteen weeks! By March I hit my goal and was at 11.6 percent body fat. But here's the real mind-blowing fact that I want to point out:

Even though I had dropped more than 12 percent body fat in four months, my body weight only dropped by five total pounds! That means if I had relied on the weight scale to tell me how I was doing, I would have completely been fooled into thinking my body wasn't making huge changes, when in fact I had dropped inches and gone from having a normal post-baby body to one that was lean and sculpted in only four months.

You must use other forms of measurement in addition to a scale to help monitor your progress. Weight is deceptive. You can actually weigh *more*, even if you're dropping body fat, because muscle weighs more than fat. But you'll still look better, feel better – and no one will know that your weight is still the same or maybe even more than it was, when you look like you lost thirty pounds!

The Cardinal Rule - Eat More Frequently

Remember when I said earlier that we have to reset your mind to think in terms of eating five small meals every day, rather than three? That's the cardinal rule to follow when you want to lose body fat and boost your metabolism. Eating five small meals a day may sound like a lot, but it's really not.

It's simply the three balanced meals you're already accustomed to, plus two snacks.

The timing of your meals is as important as the quality of the nutrition. You want your meals to be spaced at about every three to three and a half hours. Eating frequently keeps your metabolism in good order and working efficiently; studies show that it accelerates the metabolism so you can burn more calories throughout the day.

Eating frequently has other benefits as well:

- It boosts your energy levels and keeps them more consistent; stabilizes your blood sugar levels, and that means you're less likely to eat the wrong foods during the day.

- It helps you increase your concentration and mental focus.

- It reduces your food cravings and the likelihood of bingeing on the wrong foods.

- Allows for a variety of foods, which means you can more easily incorporate valuable fruits and vegetables with essential nutrients in them and space them out for better absorption in your body throughout the day.

- Keeps you fuller longer.

Here is a Sample Super Mom Fat Loss Meal Plan

1. Breakfast -- 4 egg whites + 1 starch

For me, I usually do 4 egg whites (no yolk) scrambled and 1 piece of whole-wheat toast with Smart Balance Light Butter and a little honey on top. I also have a tiny glass of skim milk with my vitamins at this meal. (I find if I take my vitamins early in the day I have the energy to take care of the kids, cook, go to the gym, and do all the things I do every single day.)

2. Mid-morning (3 hours later) -- 2 protein muffins OR an egg white protein shake

(mix 3/4 cup pasteurized liquid egg whites with 1/2 cup low sugar skim milk and 2 tablespoons Nesquik, no sugar added chocolate mix all mixed together) This shake is DELICIOUS and yields about 20 - 24 grams of protein.

3. Lunch (2 – 3 hours later) -- 4 ounces of lean meat with 3/4 cup complex carbohydrate with 1 cup vegetable

4. Mid-afternoon (2 - 3 hours later) -- 4 ounces of lean meat with 2/3 cup complex carbohydrate with 1 cup vegetable OR repeat protein shake

If you do the shake a second time, add an apple or Fage Total 0% Greek yogurt with fruit topping.

Always be sure to read the labels and try to keep sugar to under 40 grams per day.

But you do not count sugar found naturally in fruits and vegetables.

5. Dinner (3 hours later) -- 4 - 5 ounces of lean meat, DROP THE COMPLEX CARB, 2 cups of vegetables, or a dinner salad with fat free dressing

Water: Approximately 70 - 80 ounces per day

You may be asking, *"Do the portions and frequency differ based on body weight, height or desired weight loss goals?"*

Good question, and the answer is yes, but not significantly enough for you to worry so much about it that you need to come up with your own personal formula that differs from mine. Keep in mind that if you use the Rule of Thirds as provided, you're using your body's own proportions because your own hand and fist are the measuring tools. You can also use the fitness industry standard's formula for determining how much protein is required to meet your goal of gaining lean muscle mass and shedding body fat, which is to consume .8 - 1.0 grams of protein per pound of your current body weight per day.

Fit Mom Tips

Keep the grams of protein per pound of body weight to .8-1.0 if your goal is to tone, but add less muscle, and depending on your fitness and activity level. You'll still burn fat in the second scenario, but you'll likely build more muscle (which burns fat at rest), so you'll probably hit your goal quicker.

If you have a substantial amount of weight to lose, such as twenty pounds or more, then try to incorporate a cardio exercise at least three days per week for at least thirty minutes. It's true cardio won't change body shape like resistance training, but it will burn lots of calories and help you reach your goal faster.

Here's how it works:

FORMULA

Used with the permission of nutritionist Keith Klein and the Institute of Eating Management

Take your Current Body Weight x .8 – 1.0 grams of lean protein and ÷ 5 (total meals in a day) = Grams of protein required per meal

For example, let's use an average weight of 140 pounds x 1.0 = 140 ÷ 5 = 28 grams of protein per meal.

It's important to try to break out your protein consumption evenly throughout your day so your body absorbs it and uses it more efficiently.

Your body can only use a certain percentage of anything you put into it at a time. Think of the gas tank on your car and let's say it holds twenty gallons at a time. Well, if you put more in, it's simply not going to hold it or be able to use it. Your body responds the same way and when you're consuming protein you want to be sure you're consuming what you can easily absorb and burn within a three-hour period so you **maximize your potential for fat loss**. Protein is the most essential building block for creating precious muscle tissue, and the more muscle you have, the more fat you will burn. Remember, you can weigh more having more muscle on your physique, yet look smaller and thinner (leaner) because of how the muscles fill in where you had fat before.

How Food Labels Deceive You

Here are a few buying tips when shopping for lean meats. If you are still breastfeeding, when planning out your meals to assist with weight loss, keep your fat calories at 30 percent or less. If you're no longer breastfeeding and want to get more aggressive and drop more fat, keep your fat calories to under 20 percent. That's for the *entire* meal, not just for the protein. Here's an example: If you're buying ground turkey meat, make sure to get the "Extra Lean," not the "Lean.") The "Lean" version of the same product has "93/7" on the label, which leads you to believe it's 93 percent lean and only 7 percent fat, keeping your required fat intake under 20 percent. But that's simply not true. The "Lean" product is actually 41 percent fat. The "Extra Lean" ground turkey has "99/1" on the label, which suggests the product is 99 percent lean and only 1 percent fat, right?

But this product is actually 12.5 percent fat.

It's a much better product and does fulfill your goal of staying under 20 percent fat to reach your weight loss goals, but it's still 11.5 percent fat higher than the label suggested. Why is that?

The Magic Fat-Loss Formula

Total Fat Calories (sometimes written as **Total Calories from Fat**) ÷ **Calories per Serving = Percentage of Fat in Food**

To determine the percentage of fat in a food, take the Fat Calories and divide that number by the Calories Per Serving and then you'll have your Total Fat percentage.

You can take a calculator with you to the grocery store to help make your determination. My phone has one built into its Utilities.

Here's how it works. As mentioned, for fat loss, all your calories should be 20 percent fat or less. If you're unsure, look at the label on the product. Let's say the Calories Per Serving are 130 and the fat calories are 45 – if you divide 45 by 130, you come up with 0.34, which means that the product is 34 percent fat and you should avoid it.

You're probably now wondering why the actual fat percentage in the food differs so much from what the product label says. **This is because food manufacturers are allowed to print percentage of fat by WEIGHT of the product, not by actual caloric content. It's definitely buyer beware, because some manufacturers use this common misconception on the part of buyers to their advantage all the time.**

According to nutritionist Keith Klein, by adding water, binders and fillers, luncheon meat companies can make their meats appear low in fat, when they are really high in fat.

"A company can slice the meat so thin that it contains less than one gram of fat per serving," says Klein. *"So even though the label advertises the chicken is 3 percent fat by weight, it actually contains 28 percent fat by calories!"* Don't be fooled on the label by what the manufacturer gives as the "serving size." Stick to the Rule of Thirds or an actual food scale for measuring out your food and buy the foods I list here. You'll be OK if you stick with me on this.

If you buy ground beef, make sure you get the kind that is only 4 percent fat on the label – it will say "96/4" on the package. If it says "85 percent lean" or "15 percent fat," it's still actually more than 50 percent fat. The one that says "96/4" on the label is still 26 percent fat, but is still way less than the other one, which is 58 percent fat by calories. Think about this: it means the food is more than half fat!

If you can buy organic or grass fed beef, that's even better, because a lot of mass-produced meat has added hormones. And if you can only afford to buy one thing that's organic and grass fed, make it your eggs and meat products.

Lean Meats (Protein)

Boneless skinless chicken breast	Mahi-mahi
Extra lean ground turkey breast	Orange roughy*
Turkey breast	Pike
Egg whites or egg substitutes	Pollock
Cod	Red snapper
Crab	Salmon*
Flounder	Scallops
Grouper	Shrimp
Haddock	Swordfish*
Halibut	Tuna*
Mackerel*	Fat-free cottage cheese**

*Fish with asterisks contain higher levels of fat

Used with the permission of nutritionist Keith Klein and the Institute of Eating Management

Why You Should Eat Carbs

When most people think of eating carbohydrates, they usually think first in terms of bread, potatoes and pasta. But carbohydrates can be broken up into two categories – complex and simple. Those first few carbs mentioned above fall into the simple category. Simple carbs are broken down easily by the body and take a shorter period of time to digest, meaning, you won't burn as many calories digesting simple carbs because they convert to sugar so quickly. Additionally, because of their quick sugar conversion, simple carbs cause insulin spikes as a response to the resulting higher blood sugar levels, which can lead to common energy "crashes." But even though simple carbs get a bad rap, carbohydrates are a macronutrient that your body needs.

Your brain actually runs on carbohydrates – it needs a certain amount of glucose to function properly. If your body doesn't get enough of this essential "energy" macronutrient, it starts attacking itself, usually by breaking down its own muscle. And as I mentioned earlier, consuming enough protein for the body is what helps you build and maintain nice muscle.

My friends, Lee Labrada and nutritionist Keith Klein call muscle the "metabolic furnace of the body," which is to say, the more muscle you have, the more calories you burn, even at rest. The quickest way to lose body fat and lean down, the healthy way, is to build and preserve that sacred muscle tissue. In essence, carbohydrates (the good kind) are your body's running mate to losing body fat and getting into great shape. Your body needs the protein to build the muscle tissue, and it needs carbohydrates for essential energy. When you consume complex carbs (vs. simple) with a good lean protein source, you slow down the release of sugar into the blood considerably, keeping insulin levels lower and more stable. You can slow it down even more by consuming vegetables with every meal and by drinking lots of water.

Complex Carbohydrates

➡ Complex carbs can be divided into starches and vegetables. (Fruits are simple carbohydrates because of their natural sugar amounts.)

Simple Carbohydrates

*Remember to limit your consumption of sugar to less than 40 grams per day.

➡ It's important to limit processed carbs (foods made with white flour, such as pasta, breads, crackers, bagels, etc.) Simple carbs convert into sugar when your body processes them and so your body burns fewer calories during digestion.
That's why you want to shop for complex carbohydrates instead.

→ Avoid canned fruits and dried fruits because they often have loads of sugar and sodium (however in a pinch, I've used canned organic vegetables soaked in water for my kids). Studies have shown the nutrients to be just as high as fresh or frozen vegetables, but you do need to consider the packaging and whether or not the cans contain BPA or other harmful elements. Used in moderation though, I think they're fairly safe to use and definitely can be used in the Fit Mom's tool belt of super nutritious foods.

Vegetables:

Artichokes	Carrots	Lettuce
Shallots	Zucchini	Asparagus
Cauliflower	Mushrooms	Spinach
Bamboo Shoots	Celery	Okra
Spaghetti Squash	Broccoli	Eggplant
Onions	Sprouts	Brussels Sprouts
Green Beans	Peppers	Tomato
Cabbage	Leeks	Radishes
Water Chestnuts		

Fit Mom Tips

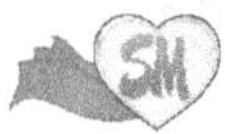 Prepare all carbs and vegetables using no butter or oil. I actually like my vegetables raw or steamed. Try Smart Balance Light, Promise Ultra Light Margarine or Fleischmann's Fat Free margarine. Top baked potatoes with a fat free dressing, salsa or ketchup.

 Rather than using water to cook vegetables, try cooking them in a fat-free chicken broth to get extra color and flavor.

 A food scale is helpful for measuring out servings until you can eyeball them, but here is a good rule of thumb:

- roughly 4 – 5 ounces of lean meat is usually the size of your palm

- roughly 3/4 cup complex carb or vegetable is the size of your fist

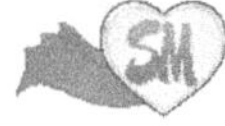 Use only fat-free salad dressings and marinades. Many of the ones that say "Light" or "Reduced Fat" on the label still contain more than 40 percent fat calories.

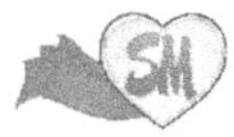 Try to consume about .8 - 1.0 gram of protein per pound of body weight.

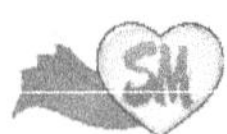 Take a calculator with you to the supermarket so you can determine the fat percentages in foods. I use my smartphone.

FIT MOM SECRET:

If you buy the gourmet cooking stock, it tends to have better flavoring than the generic or grocery-store-brand broth. Cook's Illustrated magazine recently rated the top chicken broths you can buy at the store. After testing out more than forty based on flavor, their top rated was Swanson, Certified Organic Free Range Chicken Broth, $2.79 for a 32-ounce carton.

The following listed foods are interchangeable. For example, you can substitute 3/4 cup barley or 1 serving of oatmeal for 3/4 cup rice and so on. These go on your carbohydrates list.

Interchangeable Carbohydrates

Barley	3/4 cup
Beans	3/4 cup
Black eyed peas	3/4 cup
Bread*	2 slices (*I do only one, in the morning.*) Make sure to buy the ones that are only 40 - 45 calories per slice.
Corn	3/4 cup
Corn Tortillas	2 (*I do one and then keep my lean meat serving the same at 4 ounces*)
Cream of wheat, rice or rye	3/4 cup
Kashi	3/4 cup
Lentils	3/4 cup

Oatmeal	3/4 cup
Peas	3/4 cup
Potato	6 ounces
Yam	6 ounces
Rice	3/4 cup
Rice cakes	2

Eating Healthy vs. Eating *Lean* and Healthy

When I had Luke, my second child, I had already been through the process once of having a baby and losing the baby weight. I knew what to do, and continued eating well-timed meals, organic fruits and vegetables, and eased back into my workout about four times a week. And yet, after several weeks, I was exhausted from the training, but still hadn't shed a pound. And I was working out four to five times per week! I'd worked for Labrada Nutrition, a sports nutrition company, for years, had access to amazing people in the industry who could help me, and yet I wasn't losing the rest of the baby weight and was getting frustrated. Finally, I went to my nutritionist to get some help.

> "Keith, I'm eating healthy meals, I'm doing intense workouts several times a week, and I'm still not losing the weight as fast as I think I should be."

He said, *"Tell me what you're eating, and when."* So I did. We wrote it all down and looked at it. I had been eating between three and four meals a day, spaced around my son's nap schedule and the workouts I was doing.

While it was true I had been eating *healthy* foods, Keith quickly pointed out that there's a difference between eating *healthy* and eating *lean*. Our goal was to formulate a program that had me doing *both*.

This is a really important point that a lot of people miss! They don't realize that nutrition is about 80 percent of your weight loss success and exercise is only about 20 percent. Many people over-inflate their workout and then refuel their body tank with junk it can't use to maximize weight loss.

You don't have to spend hours at the gym every day to get great results if you're feeding your body the right foods. Again, think about the efficiency your car experiences when you put in synthetic oil versus regular. You might feel it pick up a little bit more in the gear shifts; when you increase your speed, it keeps up and stays smooth.

FIT MOM SECRET:

Your body will use whatever it can to survive, but just like your car, if you give it better quality fuel so it doesn't have to work so hard, you'll feel and see the difference.

Here's a comparison of what I was eating on my own and what I switched to eating after consulting with Keith:

Meals Before

Breakfast – Three egg whites with one yolk, English muffin with butter, one cup of skim milk

Mid-morning snack – Luna Bar

Lunch – Organic quesadillas or chicken tacos, water or milk, fruit

Mid-afternoon snack – Luna Bar or Fig Newtons

Dinner – Grilled chicken and vegetables or pasta with lean beef sauce and vegetables

Meals After

Breakfast – 4 egg whites scrambled, no yolk, slice of whole grain or whole wheat bread, toast with Smart Balance Light Butter, half cup skim milk, vitamins

Mid-morning snack – Homemade protein shake (*see recipes)

Lunch – 4 ounce lean chicken breast or lean white fish, cup of vegetables, one serving of complex carbohydrates

Mid-afternoon snack – Homemade protein shake OR half of tuna sandwich OR Labrada Lean Body Shake, plus Fage 0% Greek yogurt with fruit flavoring (included in the yogurt)

Dinner – 5 ounce grilled chicken breast, vegetables, one serving of complex carbohydrates (Drop the carb at dinner to lose fat quicker)

So, what was wrong with my "before" list that kept me from losing the weight the way I wanted? Well, for one thing I wasn't eating enough before to sustain increased muscle growth, which leads to fat loss, and that meant I wasn't losing fat even with all the work I was doing. I needed to add in at least one more meal per day, do a better job with timing the meals at intervals of three to three and a half hours, and I needed to increase my protein significantly.

Additionally, the afternoon snack of a Luna Bar was an OK choice, but it was too high in sugar and wasn't helping me with the protein requirements and balancing out the Rule of Thirds with a protein source, vegetable and complex carb, so we completely reworked that snack to be more filling, more substantial, and more balanced. One of the best ways to see results right away is to make sure you don't skip meals, especially breakfast.

How to Order at a Restaurant

Even if you're doing a great job preparing and eating lean meals during the week, you can easily sabotage all your hard work if you go out to eat. My husband I enjoy being social and taking the boys out. It helps to break up the week and celebrate the weekend with something fun. But I'm also aware this is where the calories can sneak up on you because when you order out – even something seemingly harmless, like a salad – you don't know how the food was prepared or how much fat is really in the dressing.

Did they add butter or oil? Was the chicken pre-marinated, and if so, in what? Did they cook the fish in butter?

So, when I order at a restaurant I often create my own à la carte dish using ingredients I know I can eat and stay on track. If you're polite and explain you're trying to eat lean and healthy, most restaurants are happy to accommodate you. Smile real big and don't feel bad about asking for something that's going to help you. If all else fails, fall back on saying you have *special dietary needs that require you to stick to certain items*. The restaurant staff will assume this means you have an allergy or another health issue that needs to be treated carefully. And it's the truth, really, but your special health situation is that you don't want to get derailed when you're trying to accomplish your goal. But they don't need to know this.

There's nothing wrong with that, especially when you make it clear you're happy to pay for the substitutions and extra accommodations. When the restaurant gets it right, leave a big tip! They'll always be happy to serve you this way if you reciprocate by appreciating their willingness to work with you. I also make a point to return to the restaurants that are typically no hassle for me to do this, and they get more of my business and better tips.

Fit Mom Tips for Ordering at Restaurants

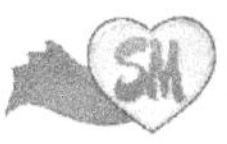 Start with a lean protein base, like chicken or fish, and find out how it's prepared.

 Ask them to grill it using no butter or oil.

 If it's been pre-marinated, sometimes they have a few pieces of meat that haven't been prepared yet, so ask for that.

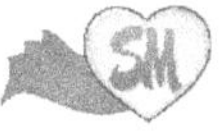 Find out what sides they have for other entrees and then request those be substituted in for yours. For example, if you see grilled or sautéed vegetables on another entrée, ask if they can add that to your meal instead of the French fries.

 If you order a side salad, which can be an excellent way to add in vegetables, ask for an oil and vinegar dressing on the side, or balsamic vinaigrette. It's even better if the restaurant offers a fat-free dressing, but most don't. You can always keep packets of fat-free dressing in your purse for such occasions, but I typically forget to do this! I find it's not an issue, though, if I stick to these other guidelines.

 If you go to a barbeque place, look for the grilled chicken or grilled chicken sandwich. Add grilled or sautéed vegetables to go with it.

 Another option at most grills is to get a baked potato with nothing on it and add four – five ounces of grilled chicken breast. Then add in your green onion, tiny amount of cheese for flavor and either salsa or a low fat sour cream. This meal is often my staple if we eat out at lunchtime during the weekend. It's satisfying, covers the Rule of Thirds, and keeps me full until my next meal, three hours later.

SECTION TWO
FITNESS AND DIET

Getting Back Into Super Shape

Getting back into shape after just having had a baby may seem impossible, but on the contrary, it is very possible – and in my opinion, highly *necessary,* in order for you to perform at your optimum level as a parent. Look at it this way: How will you possibly be able to give around-the-clock care and be at your best physically if you do not feel good; if you're limited by excess baby weight, extreme fatigue and low energy because your metabolism is thrown off? The answer is: You can do your best, but you still will not *be* at your best. So I recommend getting back into exercise as soon as you recover from the delivery.

Perhaps you don't think of yourself as being athletic. Or maybe you're not sure how soon you can begin an exercise routine with all your added responsibilities as a new Mommy. I know exactly how that last one feels! Plus, I know from personal experience that if you had a c-section, your doctor is likely going to tell you to take it easy for at least twelve weeks until your body heals. So go ahead and do that – take the time you need for your body to heal and get ready. Don't worry if you've never been athletic.

The good news about making changes in your body is you're never too old or too out of shape to begin.

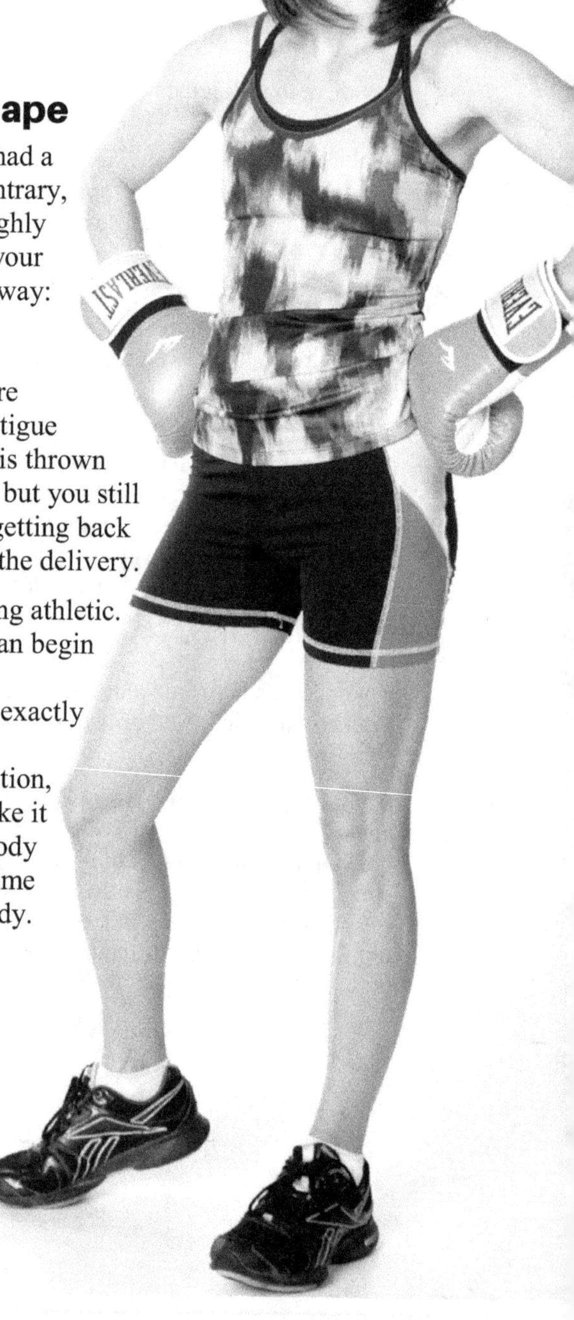

And you don't have to train like a competitive bodybuilder to make positive changes. The plan I'm going to give you will get you into excellent shape, and it's doable for a new mom, or even moms with older kids.

After this section, you will know:

➡ How to fit in gym or exercise time at home around your baby or young child's nap schedule.

➡ How to follow a pre-determined exercise plan that will maximize your results in the shortest time possible.

➡ What exercises to do at the gym that are the most effective.

➡ What tools you need to drop baby weight quickly and maintain a healthy milk supply, if you're breastfeeding.

My second pregnancy was much more difficult than the first and so I was anxious to get into the gym as soon as my doctor cleared me at my six-week follow-up appointment. I'm one of those people who doesn't feel like myself when I'm not training, but with my second pregnancy it wasn't possible for me to work out from the fourth month on – unfortunately, Luke was sitting right on top of my sciatic nerve. I ended up having to go to the chiropractor once a week for the second half of my pregnancy, just so I could get some sleep. So when I got the green light, I ran to the gym (literally!) as soon as I could.

I asked people in my local Mom's group for suggestions on a family-friendly place with childcare nearby, mentioning that it had been seven weeks since delivery and I was ready to get back in the gym as soon as possible. I did in fact receive many helpful suggestions, but one respondent actually said she thought seven weeks was way too early to even think about training! I was bewildered – for me, training was like breathing and I couldn't wait to get in there. But everybody's different. If the timing just isn't right for you and you're still adjusting to being a new mom, then listen to what you need and by all means wait until you're ready. But if you need someone to simply give you that honest girlfriend nudge so you get moving, then I'm here to do it. Get moving!

Fit Mom Responses to Your Objections!

As you're going through your closet, you'll soon realize many of your favorite clothes no longer fit and your body has changed since having kids. Realize you CAN and WILL get your shape back! But it takes time. It took you nine months to put the weight on; it will take some time to get it off again.

If your kids are already a bit older, remember it took years to put on the weight you want to lose. Give yourself some time and some grace! With consistency, you WILL get there.

But remember, after following the diet plan and workout regimen I'm giving you, I was able to go from 26 percent body fat to 14 percent body fat within 4 months. Four months is nothing!

That's one season out of the year and you can be back in shape, or even better! So you can definitely reach your goals with persistence and consistency – and even within a shorter period of time than you may have imagined.

Right now I'm hearing the objections formulate in your mind. But you have to ask yourself, *how badly do I want this?* Only you can decide. But I promise you, the minute you make the decision to change your body, if you stick with this program, you'll soon be in amazing shape.

Here are some common Mom Objections that I know may be filling your mind, and my Fit Mom responses:

1. **I had a c-section and my doctor still hasn't cleared me to exercise.**
   Typically, your ObGyn will tell you to wait twelve weeks before exercising after a c-section, but in many cases you can begin sooner. You need to tell your doctor what kinds of exercises you'd like to start doing, and as long as the stitches have healed internally, you should get the OK to begin a light- to medium-intensity training program. Stay away from too much abdominal work, and for very high-intensity stuff, such as kickboxing and some forms of strenuous core moves, like push-ups, it's best to wait the full twelve weeks while all the abdominal muscle layers heal. You'll also want to avoid isolating abdominals until the layers of muscle from your surgery have completely healed, and the timing varies per individual, so that's the reason why most physicians will say to play it safe.

2. **My baby is too young to take to the gym with me.**
   Many gyms offer childcare for babies beginning as early as six weeks old. The YMCA is one of them, and you can check around for others in your area. I recommend checking out the gym and nursery ahead of time so you're comfortable. Find out what the nursery staff is able to do for your baby, whether it's offering a bottle or rocking to sleep or just playing while you work out, so you can determine the best time to take your little one with you. If you've read *Secrets of the Super Moms, Part I,* you'll remember that I recommend doing this around your baby's schedule so you can keep the routine you've worked so hard to achieve with him. For example, I would never take a baby to the gym during naptime, but if it's a snack or mealtime, perhaps the nursery caregiver can feed the

baby for you while you're working out. However, if you're uncomfortable taking your baby with you until he or she is older, this program is also designed for you to be able to work out at home while your baby naps. See the **Workout in a Box**, stick with it, and you'll still get results and be better off than if you just skipped the gym.

And remember, I offer a comprehensive at-home fitness program with community support, accountability, and motivational tools to keep you on track. If you want more personalized guidance, check it out at *www.FitMomSecrets.com/Book-Offer*

3. **I'm still breastfeeding and I'm not sure how to make that work with my exercise schedule.**
   With both of my kids I found I was able to get in a full workout and have more time to myself if I planned my workouts around their needs. For example, go ahead and nurse your baby at home (or in the ladies restroom at your gym if you're comfortable), and then bring your baby to the gym with you during his or her **Wake / Play Time**. Your baby will be happier, more alert, and you will buy yourself enough time for a full training session. You'll want to make sure you still have enough support for your breasts by wearing a nursing sports bra, and keep in mind you'll have a much better workout and be more comfortable anyway, after you've emptied your breasts from your baby's meal.

   I've seen babies in the nursery when it's normally their naptime – they're exhausted, and quite understandably, irritable. The nursery staff has to work that much harder to get them to settle down and be content until their mommies come back. In my opinion, it's much better to meet your baby's feeding and nap needs first, then you'll have a better chance at getting that training time you need. Plus, you'll feel like a better mom in the process. With breastfeeding, it takes a little extra planning, but it's still doable. And if you're still not sure or not comfortable, all the exercises offered here can be done at home. Check out the **Workout in a Box Section**.

4. **I need to eat an additional 500 calories per day to produce good breast milk. Should I do it all at once or space it out over the course of the day?**
   Five hundred calories may sound like a lot, but it really isn't. It's also the minimum number of additional calories you might need now if you're breastfeeding. Some women need more, and that's entirely an individual thing. But start with 500 and add more if you find you're still not producing enough milk for your baby. You can easily eat an additional 500 to support your milk production without going overboard and sabotaging your training program.

Consider this: 500 calories = one extra chicken breast, one banana, two egg whites and an eight-ounce glass of skim milk. My suggestion is to space this food out over your five meals you're consuming anyway. For example, you can add an extra egg white or two in the morning with your breakfast, cut up the chicken breast and space out between your lunch and dinner so you can finish it. Then add in the banana during your mid-morning or mid-afternoon snack.

You could add the skim milk to a protein shake or drink at breakfast with your vitamins. Also, consider adding in an Omega 3 supplement to get in added essential fats.

FIT MOM SECRET:

Our bodies are typically drained after a good workout session anyway, so you might also bump up the protein you consume immediately after your workout (like a protein shake you prepared in advance and brought with you to the gym) to keep your milk production strong for your baby's next meal.

And definitely drink lots of water. Start sipping on it early in the day right after breakfast and make sure to refill your water jug before you go to the gym and do a class or go to the weight room. The extra water will help to support your breast milk production.

5. **I'm so incredibly exhausted – more so than when I had a full time career. More so than ever before!**

Yes, being a new mother is exhausting! You're expected to be on call around the clock, and often, what's being demanded is the breast milk you spent the day producing. And all you want to do is sleep – because your little one isn't yet. Well, working out and eating five meals a day will kick-start your metabolism again. The more muscle you build, the more fat you will burn. And simultaneously you'll feel energized and excited to know you're making good changes in your body. Pretty soon, you'll start to see it and the clothes that were too snug during your pregnancy and then after you had your baby, will start to fit again. This is an exciting time in your life! And then it gets even better: around twelve weeks your little one will start extending his nighttime sleep, and that means Mama gets more sleep, too. The workout is critical for regaining your energy, and it will happen!

When we work out our brains release "feel good" hormones, called endorphins, that boost our mood and energy levels. It's like the first time you and your spouse started dating and you felt happy all the time.

Well, you can create that by exercising and stimulating the release of those hormones naturally on a daily basis. It's actually how you can *add more time* to your day even by taking the time out to exercise.

You feel better, you're happier and therefore more productive, which equals more Super You to spread around. Exercise also can add *years to your life* and increase your quality of life and what you have to give your children. Don't feel guilty about taking care of yourself so you can take care of your children and serve others. It's important!

6. **Will I sabotage my breast milk supply by training too early?**
   To be perfectly honest, that can happen, and it was one of my concerns before I began working out again. That's why it's so important to not only consume the right balance of foods as outlined in the previous section, but to also make sure they are in the right proportions. If you're breastfeeding, make sure to consume <u>at least</u> 500 more calories to fuel your body with the right nutrients to offset the extra calories you're burning in the workout. You'll know within a week or so if your milk supply is suffering. And it's possible you might have to supplement with formula at one of your baby's meals or increase your calories a little more until you find the right balance. It's a delicate act – I know; I've been there. My best advice is to start off slow with the training.

   Focus more on the resistance than the cardio if you feel like your milk supply is suffering because of it. You can always add in more cardio later when you're no longer breastfeeding. For a more exact recommendation on which calories to consume, how much and when, contact me directly on my public Facebook page at *Facebook.com/SecretsOfTheSuperMom* and I'm happy to connect you to my nutritionist directly.

7. **I have even less time now, because of my baby's schedule, and I want to spend that time with my family.**
   For you, the best time of day to get in your workout is probably before your baby wakes up. If it helps you, this program can also be broken down into two shifts. For example, you can break the thirty-minute routine into two fifteen-minute routines. Just keep your Workout in a Box set up from the prior session, and during the baby's second nap, squeeze in that second session.

That way, by the time your entire family is home together, you can all be together and know you've already done the workout. Enjoy your time with your family.

8. **I just don't know where to fit it into my schedule.**
   This program is flexible, so try it out at different times of the day and see what works best for you. Remember, as your baby's schedule and routine changes, you'll adjust yours likewise. So in the beginning weeks, maybe the best time to fit it in is during the morning and mid-day naps, spaced out in two sessions. As your baby gets older, you can do it at the gym or keep it going at home, and just work around things as needed.

FIT MOM SECRET:

One thing I've learned from being a mother is that if I don't SCHEDULE and PLAN my time like an appointment on the calendar, everyone else's agenda gets met before mine.

But if I keep certain items as standing appointments on my calendar, i.e., my workouts, then I find I can fit in my training sessions and still carve out time to do other things, whether it's a work project, meeting someone at the house for scheduled maintenance, lunch with friends, running errands, writing or taking time to read to my son's class.

9. **I have a long commute, and by the time I get home I want to spend that time with my kids.**
   You could join a gym near your office and do these workouts during your lunch hour – that way when you get home, you're already done and don't have to fit it in around your family time. Some employers have flex time available, so in that case, you could pick the best time of day to block out your training routine where it won't inhibit your work schedule. And some companies will sponsor or pay for their employees' gym membership fees as an added perk.

   Do some research through your company's human resources department to find out if that's offered. And if not, perhaps you could be the trailblazer who helps create a company-wide get in shape health initiative.

I know it sounds like a lot to fit in a family, full time job, and working out, but the truth is, building in exercise time *creates* time for you and your family because it adds to your quality of life, longevity and energy levels.

It really is worth it if you can make it work. Do what you can. Our bodies were made to move. Training two or three times a week instead of four or five is better than not training at all. The program is flexible, so if you need to break it up into 25- or 35-minute shifts, you can.

As your child gets older, he or she can do exercises with you and you'll be starting your child on a lifelong path of interest in and understanding of the importance of taking care of the body.

10. **I travel for my job. How can I maintain this program while I'm on the road?**
    It's easier than you think! In terms of when to fit it in while traveling, it will depend on your exact schedule, but if you know you'll have a long day that's going to end late, do the workout first thing in the morning. If you have time to go back to your hotel in between projects, do it then. Remember, I offer a comprehensive Super Mom Get Fit Program that will walk you through what to do, and when, with fully interactive how-to videos, healthy recipes, eating clean journal, daily workout log, and more. It's super convenient because you can literally log in from any device, hit "Play" and work out with me! And it's very affordable. Check it out here: *www.FitMomSecrets.com/Book-Offer*.

    Many hotels have gyms in them, so before you book your work trip, make sure to book with a hotel that does have gym access or one nearby. You could possibly call ahead and ask the hotel management if you can borrow a set of dumbbells in your room for the duration of your stay in case you need to work out outside of their normal gym hours. If the hotel doesn't have a gym in it, ask the concierge for the nearest one to where you're staying and ask if they have any free guest passes. Some fitness centers have reciprocal arrangements with gyms in other cities, so call ahead and ask. And make sure to pack a set of workout clothes and shoes so you're prepared to hit the ground running, or lifting, once you arrive at your destination.

11. **I don't have a gym near my home.**
    That's OK! All the exercises in this program can be done at home just as easily and with amazing results. Here's that link again in case you'd like to check out my Super Mom Get Fit Program: *www.FitMomSecrets.com/Book-Offer*.

12. **I can't afford a gym membership.**

    You don't need a gym membership to make this program work for you. All of the exercises can be modified using at-home equipment that includes various weighted dumbbells, barbell, bench with risers, resistance band, inflatable exercise ball, and an exercise mat. Notice the notes and modifiers within for a great at-home workout that will get you the same results as the machines.

13. **I don't know where to begin or what to do to get my body back.**

    First make sure you're clear from your doctor to begin exercising. If you delivered vaginally without complications, you can potentially begin the next day if you want to! Assuming you're healthy and ready, just follow the steps in the program. It's as easy as that. The workouts are spaced to maximize the results on the muscle, so every day is planned with thought and supports the day before and the day after it. Just follow the plan and you'll see linked-in recipes and other tips to support whatever day you happen to be doing. Check out the Super Mom Get Fit Program: *www.FitMomSecrets.com/Book-Offer*.

When to Stop

Before beginning an exercise program of any kind, please get the approval of your physician.

Once you've gotten the clean bill of health and green light from your doctor, there are still a few things to watch out for when you begin training. If you notice any of these things happening, it's time to stop and listen to your body. Headaches can be a symptom that you're dehydrated, or that your head went below your heart too soon afterwards without a cool down, or that you weren't breathing properly and restricted oxygen to your brain (called the Valsalva maneuver). Exercise places great oxygen demands on your body's organs and muscles.

To meet these requirements, your blood pressure and heart rate temporarily increase while exercising to move a greater amount of oxygen to your brain and other organs within a short period of time. When you drop your head lower than your heart while your heart rate is still up, the increased blood flow can pool inside your head, which can cause headaches.

So, if you're new to exercise you might notice some weird things happening. Take a break and start the next day if:

➡ You feel nauseated. It's normal; your body is probably purging some toxins, but you should still back off.

➡ You feel sick.

⇒ You have cold sweats or chills.

⇒ You suddenly go pale or can't catch your breath after a five-minute rest.

⇒ You have a very painful and concentrated headache.

Take the initial rest you need and then resume the following day. If the symptoms persist it's time to talk to your doctor about it and see if there is an underlying issue, like perhaps you're getting sick and didn't realize it. (If you are getting sick, take the rest and recovery days you need, otherwise you could make it worse.)

Success Secrets

At times, even the most dedicated athletes need inspiration to push themselves to the next level. You're only human if you have to give yourself a pep talk every now and then to stick with it. My iPhone has an alarm at 9 a.m. every single day and includes one of my built-in affirmations: *"Eat clean and you can do it!"* It might seem silly, as though it should be easy for a disciplined person like me to do the steps daily that get positive results, but believe me, I'm just like anyone else and I have to tell myself to do it.

My one advantage is that I have the benefit of knowing if that I do "X" for long enough, I'll get the "Y" results I'm aiming for, because I've already gone through this process a few times.

Here are some of the pep talks I give myself that I've learned over time. Believe me, I am not trivializing your situation…I know only too well that it's not an easy feat to go to the gym with a baby or toddler and remember everything you need to bring with you. Because of course that will be the moment when your child starts protesting putting on shoes and cries the minute he sees the nursery room. Hang in there, Super Mom!

FIT MOM SECRET #1:

Focus on the positive. Don't think to yourself, "Nothing I could wear before fits me. I feel so big and sloppy." Think this instead: "While my clothes don't fit me now, I can get back to size X by June 20."

FIT MOM SECRET #2:

Set your goals in 4-, 8-, or 12-week increments to give yourself positive motivation. It's much easier to tackle any major endeavor when you break it up into chunks rather than trying to visualize the entire journey all at once. Case in point: writing this book!

FIT MOM SECRET #3:

Tell others about your plan so they will encourage you. When you let your friends know what your goals are they will support you and cheer you on. It's also a great idea to get a gym buddy or meet someone in a class who knows to look for you on the specific days you attend.

You'll begin to support one another and if for whatever reason one of you misses, the other will notice and follow up. Look for ways that you can be an encourager, too.

FIT MOM SECRET #4:

Set your mind. Tell yourself, every day, with every meal, *"I am eating this lean, healthy meal because I want a lean, fit body."* Remember why you're doing it so you can keep going on the tough days, and believe me, there will tough days where you just have to get to the gym when you don't want to, or it's raining, and when you want to eat something greasy and fried. Refrain!

I promise, your reward in just a few short weeks will be your beautiful, lean physique and you'll have so much energy and feel so great, you won't even remember that gross hamburger that nearly derailed you.

Get more personalized support in my Super Mom Get Fit Program: *www.FitMomSecrets.com/Book-Offer*.

FIT MOM SECRET #5:

Pull out the things you want to wear but can't right now and put them in a place where you'll have a visual reminder of your goal every day. Look through magazines and pull out a photo of someone who has a similar build or body type as you, and who has a physique you admire. Put the photo of that person (or it could be you from an earlier time in your life) on your bathroom mirror so you'll have that clear image in your head every time you wake up and get ready. Be very clear on what you want to accomplish and don't look back. Victory will be yours within WEEKS!

FIT MOM SECRET #6:

Recognize no one just wakes up with a naturally beautiful and perfect physique. No one. Not even athletes. It takes a great deal of determination and hard work. But here's the secret no one ever tells you: **You have the power to achieve this for yourself!** Despite genetics, your preconceptions about yourself, your past bad eating habits, partying too much in college, too many happy hours – you can still create a healthy, lean body. I'm here to help you get there .

FIT MOM SECRET #7:

Think of yourself as already being the person you want to be. You have to think and train like an athlete to be an athlete. One thing that really helps me to get into that mindset is to find inspiring transformation stories of others who were once overweight and who have completely changed their lives with diet and nutrition. They are everywhere!

You can search inside popular fitness magazines like *Oxygen, Fitness, Women's Health, People* or you can watch *The Biggest Loser* on NBC, *Joy Bauer's Fit Club* on the *Today Show*, or look at the "wall of fame" at your gym for pictures of people who were once very overweight and decided to make a change.

When you look at people who are in incredible shape, and who are lean, toned, fit and energetic – all the things you want to be – it's tempting to think that it just happened overnight. Or that maybe they were just born that way.

Certainly, genetics do play a small role.

However, when I saw some of the success stories at Labrada Nutrition, and witnessed some of my friends overcome tremendous obstacles, like breast cancer, fibromyalgia, and negative body image and find the lean person they had inside – despite genetics and having not grown up in healthy households where lean foods were a priority – I was incredibly inspired.

That taught me that those results could be possible for anybody, regardless of their physical condition.

I've seen the evidence for myself: My nutritionist's office walls are peppered with signed photographs from his clients, profusely thanking him for their amazing results.

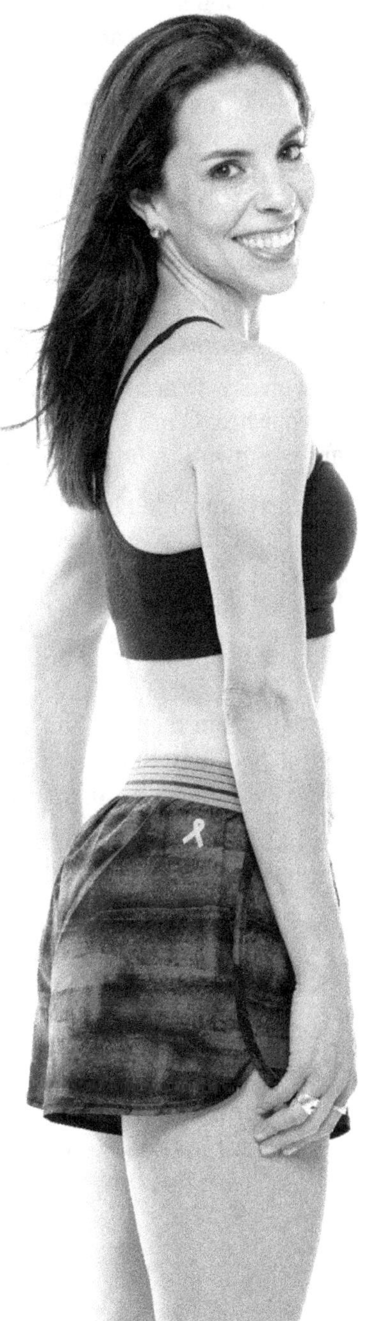

We've all seen *The Biggest Loser* on NBC, where people lose 100-plus pounds – of course, that particular situation is accomplished by extreme conditioning in order to provide entertainment for television viewers, but the results are still obtainable. It bears repeating – despite genetics, people can overcome tremendous things and do, every day. You can be one of them!

So when you think about yourself and consider what you want in life, think about the lean person that's inside, and follow that dream. I say this here, with emphasis, because **it may never have occurred to you that you *could* have the fit and lean body you desire**. That's why I find **Fit Mom Secret #6** so revolutionary. It's possible *nobody has ever told you*, so I'm telling you now, as your friend. You can do it. And I will help you.

Staying Positive Is Vital

It's not enough to simply keep your eye on the goal, because there are so many negative messages and images pursuing and consuming our brains all the time. Your goals of finding and sculpting a lean and fit body, however noble and realistic, may not be achievable if the messages you contain within yourself are in conflict with your desired result.

It's important to know this up front and to **set your mind for a positive outcome**.

Put only positive messages into your mind and hang out with positive people who will reinforce those messages and the goals you have for yourself. Cut out the naysayers! It may be hard at first, but you will quickly recognize who ison board with you and who isn't.

The ones who aren't will only hold you back if you let them continue to be prominent in your life. Don't listen to them. Follow your dreams, because they are possible. They are worthwhile, and they are important.

You're bombarded by advertisements all the time – billboards on TV, commercials at night around 9 p.m., after you've had dinner and the kids are in bed – tempting you, nudging you, to get that "last" bite of ice cream, to have one more beer, to make buttered popcorn. And the ads say things like, *"You deserve a break, have a beer!"*

They deliberately use words like "you deserve this" and "you deserve that." "This Bud's for You! Because You're Worth It!" *Thanks, that sounds like a great idea!* And so, again, our thoughts fail us, because the commercials make us feel like we're entitled to these things, and we should have them. Only they bring us further away from our real goals, to be healthy and happy.

I'd like to position this in a different way. Certainly, yes, you do deserve those things, but let's turn that around. You *deserve* to have a lean, healthy body.

> **You deserve healthy foods, you deserve to feel and look great, your body deserves to be given the best nutrition possible so that it can sustain you during everything you'll need to go through to chase after kids, maintain a strong, healthy family, manage your career goals, and to keep your energy level up so you can be the caregiver that you need to be for your children. *That's* what you deserve...all that and more.**

Am I tempted by those relentless messages that want to lead me away from my goals? Of course, I'm only human! But then I remind myself, *I am an athlete. I want more than this cheeseburger can offer me. I train and eat like a Fit Mom. I am a lean, physically fit mother of two who must set a good example.* Sometimes I have to psych myself up to reset my mind in a positive direction and turn away from the many temptations around me. But it works, and you can do this, too.

Small Changes Add Up to Big Results

Here's something important for you to know…**once you start making small changes every day, then the choices become easier and easier until they eventually become realistic and natural for you, and you no longer have to think consciously about them all the time.** Ordering chicken breast at a restaurant without butter or oil has become second nature to me now.

I'd love to indulge in the pasta, but I know it won't help me achieve my goals, so I go for the better choice with steamed vegetables on the side.

FIT MOM SECRET #8:

Exercise and nutrition go hand in hand. You can't simply do one without the other and expect the results you want. You have to eat several lean healthy meals throughout the day and exercise at a decent intensity level to get your body to respond. The ideal timeframe to train for cardio is for about forty-five minutes with your target heart rate between 75 to 85 percent of its maximum.

To determine your ideal heart rate during cardio, take the number 180 and subtract your age. If you're 35 years old, your ideal heart rate is 180 – 35 = 145 beats per minute. I usually pick a favorite class and go do my cardio that way.

For example, on either Tuesdays or Thursdays (cardio days for me), I can attend turbo kickboxing, or I can run outside, or run intervals on the treadmill.

To determine what your intensity level should be for resistance training, you simply need to keep the movement at a slow and steady pace, keeping the tension on the muscle you're working the entire time. Complete your first set, rest for one minute, then perform your next set and so on.

For each exercise rep (repetition) you perform, inhale during the exercise and exhale at the highest point of exertion. See my workout planner later in the chapter for more details.

FIT MOM SECRET #9:

Keep a food journal and write down everything you eat in that one place. *Everything.* You must become aware of everything that goes into your mouth. How many times have you snacked on your child's remaining few Goldfish and not counted them? I've done it, too!

We don't want to waste the food we give our babies and so often we eat the left-overs off their plates ourselves.

But keeping a food journal will let you see plain and clear where your weak points are and you'll be less likely to indulge in those little cheats if you know you have to write them down!

Another trick is to write down your meals and workouts for the day before you consume and complete them because it's a written intention of what is yet to come.

By the act of putting it all down on paper, you're already setting your mind to accept those meals and commit to that workout, and you're way more likely to follow through and actually do it all. You've made a very real written contract with yourself.

FIT MOM SECRET #10:

Every single choice you make either advances you toward your goal or moves you backward away from it. There is no in-between. Remember that when your friends invite you to a happy hour for cocktails and fatty chips.

Still go and be social, by all means! But instead of snacking on the chips, move the basket aside and out of your reach.

Pretend it's not even there. Instead of ordering a sugary alcoholic beverage, get iced tea with lemon.

Ask for a pretty umbrella if it makes you feel better. You can still indulge, but be strategic about it, like on one day during the weekend when you have a glass of wine or a margarita you've been looking forward to all week. You can get back into shape within twelve weeks if you want to, but it's up to you to prepare and consume the lean meals and get in the workouts I'm presenting here.

I promise, just get started and it will get easier with time. At least I've taken all the guesswork out of it for you!

Question: *What happens if I follow your suggestions but I fall off the wagon? How do I reset myself?*

Answer: We're all human and we all experience this, even the most dedicated athletes and fitness professionals. We all go through it. My nutritionist recommends when you first start out on the nutrition program to allow yourself one cheat meal every week. This is one meal per week where you let yourself have anything you want, and then you get right back on track with the next meal.

My suggestion is to plan this in during a weekend, like on a Saturday night, so you can enjoy something fun and social with your family and do it guilt-free. Psychologically, this can be enough for many people, especially if they're the type who, when told things like, *"You can't have this,"* immediately want that thing even more – and go to great lengths to get it, even if it's damaging to their goals and what they've set out to accomplish.

The reason why I didn't focus much on the cheat meal idea is because I think it can be a slippery slope, unless you really do have the self-discipline to get right back on track afterwards and stay there.

Here's what you have to do:

Tell yourself to focus on all the great foods you can have and not on the ones you want to limit, because the psychology that goes into using the positive form of language with a toddler to get him to respond positively, is the same mind trick that works on our brains when we want to reach a goal.

We might be all grown up now but our brains still work the same way they always did! If you feel the pressure building up to the point where you think you're about to blow it all with one meal, then allow yourself a cheat meal. You probably do really need it to let off some of that internal steam. Go ahead and get a hamburger or a chocolate shake or margarita – whatever it is that you want. Go ahead and indulge, but have your next lean meal ready and waiting, so all you have to do is eat it.

One thing I do is keep some hard candy in my desk drawer or in the pantry, so in a pinch, if I want something sweet that won't derail my efforts, I'll have a little piece. Sometimes I'll have a Starburst or a small piece of chocolate, a small pacifier that tells my body, *"OK, you've had your fun, now go back to work!"* My body listens, is grateful, and we're all happy. (Certain times of the month and hormone fluctuations can trigger this, as well.)

FIT MOM SECRET #11:

Have a cheat meal occasionally. My nutritionist says one per week is OK, but my advice is to keep trying to push yourself so you don't have to give in that frequently. Lengthen the time in between…first every week, then every two weeks, then three and so on. I'm at the point now where I can go for about a month before I need to cave in. This kind of discipline takes time to develop, though, so don't feel badly if you need a cheat meal every week to begin with. Remember, it's all about progress and reaching that next mini-goal.

The Workout

Break your week out over the course of seven days and aim to fit in a minimum of three – four workouts per week. If you can fit in five, that's even better, but you also want to try to fit in at least two rest days in the week, which is why I don't recommend six – seven workouts per week. You can do all of the workouts during the week or two during the week and two over the weekend, but you need to schedule in recovery days. Resistance training tears your muscles down; it's the recovery time that builds them back up, so rest days are not optional. They are necessary for consistent results.

Some of the ladies at my gym are there every single day of the workweek and they do multiple classes on those days – sometimes two to three, back-to-back fifty-five minute classes!

But it's not necessary to work out for two or three consecutive hours every day to get results, and this type of overtraining exhausts your body and prevents it from performing properly.

And worse, it can lead to serious injury. In fact, you can begin to burn precious muscle tissue if you push too hard for too long. Work out at a high intensity for the forty-five – fifty-five minutes on the days you train, but also take at least two days each week to allow your body to recover. It's best to space out your recovery days for the best effect and not take them back to back.

Here is a sample week for how you might break up muscle groups:

- **Monday** – Back and biceps, abs
- **Tuesday** – Chest and triceps
- **Wednesday** – Rest
- **Thursday** – Legs
- **Friday** – Cardio
- **Saturday** – Back and biceps
- **Sunday** – Rest

P.S. — The Super Mom Get Fit Program is already structured like this. *www.FitMomSecrets.com/Book-Offer*

In order to get in all the major muscle groups it's important to divide them up into three distinct categories and days. This makes it easier to work them all in and supports a balanced training approach which will contribute to a more proportional and symmetrical look.

Back and biceps are ***pull*** muscles, or muscles you train by pulling them *toward* your body.

Opposing muscle groups – like chest, shoulders and triceps – are *push* muscles, or muscles you train by pushing *away* from your body. And the largest muscle group, the *kick and crunch* muscles, include the legs, abdominals and calves.

On Day One, you'll start with the pull muscles, back and biceps. On Day Two, you'll continue with the push muscles, chest and triceps, and so on through the entire first week, making sure to take rest days in between at least two days each week.

If you want to burn a little more fat, you can add one more cardio day at the beginning, either in the morning of one of your muscle group days or in place of one of your rest days, but not both.

After you've cycled through one week alternating muscle groups as shown, you'll begin the routine again, but make sure to vary the exercises each time and change the stimulus on the muscle so you effect change.

I've included a twelve-week workout plan in this book so you can see how to vary the exercises on a regular basis and still get the changes you want. You can keep repeating the twelve-week program or you can mix and match any of the exercises presented. Add in some of your own if you like.

Changing It Up

Changing the stimulus on the muscle simply means that you change your exercises and routines each time you work out so your body doesn't adapt to the point where it no longer responds. And you should alternate between using dumbbells for your exercises and using the barbell with weights or plates, because even that slight change, although it's still basically the same exercise with the same reps, can change your range of motion and hit the muscle differently.

The fun thing is that the larger your baby or toddler gets, the more he or she can be an added tool to your gym as well! I'll show you some great Mommy & Me exercises later on if your child is still young enough for them.

You Won't Look Like a Man!

Many women are fearful that they will look like men if they lift heavy. **This is a myth!** This is a very important point to address because of how deeply entrenched this fear can be…I know because early on I was one of those women! I was very concerned that if I lifted heavy – say using twelve-pound dumbbells on my shoulders (twenty-four pounds) or fifteen-pound dumbbells on my back (thirty pounds) – that it would somehow change my body's chemistry and I would morph into looking like a man!

Ladies, I can assure you that this won't happen. We are just not built to look like men. We are not built genetically to look like men, and we do not carry the same testosterone levels as a man, so we are simply not capable of developing the same physique as a man. In order to get anywhere close, we'd have to deliberately take hormones or supplements to change our body chemistry. All the weight training in the world won't turn our women's muscles into a man's muscles. Lifting to challenge our bodies with heavier weights will simply stimulate our metabolism and strengthen the muscles we have so that they become fat burning engines. And pretty soon we'll get the muscle tone we want…and curves in all the right places.

Group Weight Training

One strategy I used successfully as a new mom and recommend for you is to ***attend group weight training as you're trying to ease back into exercise***. It's a huge help for new moms to go to a class, because the instructor has already done all the planning for you and it's their job to structure the workout and think through the opposing muscles to hit the full body. This is another reason why I created the Super Mom Get Fit Program: *www.FitMomSecrets.com/Book-Offer*, to help moms with a proven plan that takes the guesswork out of training for you.

All you have to do is show up and follow instructions, and that can be an enormous relief. I know when I was a new mom that I was really grateful not to have to think about one more thing on top of everything else I was dealing with. My mind was already crammed full with figuring out when my baby was going to eat, when he was going to nap, if I needed to allow time to pump, and if I was going to fit in my workout for the day, how that workout was going to happen...and so on. I just didn't need to have to plan and structure a workout on top of all that in order to make the big changes in my body that I wanted.

Fit Mom Tips

Go as heavy as you can when weight training in group classes. The caveat to this is that keeping good form throughout the exercise is even more important than the amount of weight you're lifting. It's better to do a slightly lighter weight and keep good form than miss your position and injure yourself because the weight is too heavy. If you choose to do group classes, the instructor of your class should help you with form and posture. The reason this is important is that if the weight is too heavy you could injure yourself. However, don't allow yourself to become afraid of that and use it as an excuse to not challenge yourself. Many women fear using too large a weight or simply don't know how to choose the correct weight for various muscle groups, and they default to lifting weights that are too light for them. How can you tell? If you're able to go through a set of twelve reps with no problem and it's just a little difficult, that weight is too light for you and you're not going to get the changes in your body that you really want. It's very important that you're constantly challenging yourself, because if you do, you'll see those changes within a very short period of time. My own story is proof that it can happen within just twelve – sixteen weeks, especially if you're eating right.

If it becomes easier and you've been using the same weights for two - three months, it's time to step up the weight level. Even if the instructor is changing the workout, if you're finding it easy, then that's your cue that you definitely need to increase your weights. Again, for more personalized attention and support, go to this link: *www.FitMomSecrets.com/Book-Offer.*

The last three reps of each set should be difficult, but not impossible. How difficult? You should really have to exert yourself on the exhale as you come up in a chest press, shoulder press or squat, but know at the same time that you're not engaging the other smaller muscles around it, that you're really focused on the muscle itself. Exert yourself, yes, but it shouldn't be impossible. And remember the most important thing – you should be able to maintain your form the entire time.

One thing that can be frustrating is that sometimes your larger muscles can handle the weight, but not the smaller, connecting muscles. For example, when I'm doing chest presses, I frequently have to "drop down" my weights during the second set because my forearms start to hurt in the required wide grip, and the pain is too great for me to push the chest muscles as much as I'd like. Again, the most important thing: making progress and preventing an injury is much better than having to sit out for six weeks while you recover because you didn't listen to your body.

The power of exertion should be on the muscle itself and you shouldn't have to pull in the shoulder muscles or neck muscles when you really want to focus on just the chest or shoulder, for example. If you're having to involve too many muscles to make it through a rep or you find yourself compromising your form (your shoulders are coming up, you're shrugging to lift the weight, you can't go deep into a squat, etc.), then the weight is too heavy and you should drop the next set down.

Modification is OK! I'm a regular at a popular weight training class that's choreographed. The benefit to this type of resistance training is they fit in more reps and stimulate the muscles in all different ways during the frequent tempo changes. But there's one exercise this particular class tends to favor, and I'm opposed to it. It's the Clean and Press. I injured myself weeks ago doing this exercise, so now when everyone else in class is doing it, I simply keep the tempo and do two-arm bent-over rows. When they get back to the next exercise, I'm right there with them!

The instructor even complimented me one day for doing this because she knew it was my way of trying to avoid serious injury. Instructors don't mind it when you do this in class, and if you explain ahead of time they will often help you find a suitable alternative that helps you hit the same muscles.

Form

Proper form is extremely important. You can lift a lighter weight with excellent form and still hit the muscle in a way that is very effective. I know that sounds like I'm contradicting what I just said about the necessity to push yourself, but the point I'm making here is that focus, really thinking about what you're doing, is what counts most of all. Don't just think, *"Well, if I just go to these classes and do the movements then I can go through the motions, get it done, and my body's going to do the work for me."* That won't fly.

I know you've heard the phrase from athletes, *"It's a mental game."* It's true. When you're weight training, it's just as much mental as it is physical. You're counting, thinking about your breathing – what are you doing on the inhale, what are you doing on the exhale – concentrating on everything being in alignment and having proper form. The mirrors you see *everywhere* in a gym are so you can watch yourself…but not just to admire your cute workout gear! What you need to be watching is that your posture and form are correct.

Use your instructor as a gauge to help you determine if you're doing it right. Most of the trainers in my classes are pretty good about stressing the importance of good form. But I've also noticed many instructors don't walk around and point things out that need to be changed – it's possible that they are reluctant to embarrass anyone or make them feel uncomfortable. Unfortunately, that reluctance can be very dangerous and lead to injuries. Make it clear to your instructor that you want to be told if your form isn't correct.

Another thing to keep in mind, especially if you do attend group classes: **changing the weight format from the dumbbells to the barbell or vice versa can restrict your range of motion to focus the tension on the muscles differently**. Even changing the grip during an exercise can have a significant impact on tensing and working the muscle.

If there are any exercises that compromise your movement in any way, stop, and go back to the other format or it can increase your injury risk.

There are some exercises that are higher risk than others, and for those reasons I've listed them below as ones to avoid. For example, I injured my wrist doing the Clean and Press – the restrictive movement of performing an upright row with a heavy barbell loaded up for my legs and then catching to do the upward press put too much strain on my wrists. I didn't know this until later when I was doing Dolphin Planks and came down too hard on my already compromised and weakened wrist. By then it was too late. I couldn't bend my wrist backward, even slightly, for about six weeks. And I had to wear a wristguard to keep it immobilized so I could resume exercising.

Even a traditional grip versus a reverse grip on the same exercise can cause you to stress the muscle differently to get it to respond.

It's important to know this in advance and this is also why I've structured the **Advanced Twelve-Week Workout** the way I have – you'll notice when we do certain muscle groups, we switch from dumbbells to the barbell, and we change grips from week-to-week so you get a balanced program that activates the muscles differently every time to make them respond. As I've said before, changing up your workout on a regular basis is how you continue to make progress.

Exercises to Avoid

Sources: The Aerobics and Fitness Association of America and The American College of Sports Medicine

- ✖ **Clean and Press** (or Clean and Jerk)
- ✖ **Machine Leg Extensions**
- ✖ **Good Mornings**
- ✖ **Barbell Bent-Over Rows**
- ✖ **Barbell Upright Rows**
- ✖ **Behind-the-Neck Lat Pulldowns**
- ✖ **Smith Machine Squats and Lunges**
- ✖ **Certain compound movements to tempo**

Remember:

- ➡ Proper form is the most important thing.

- ➡ Make sure you have the right weight for you, and for the right muscle group or body part.

- ➡ Change up the workouts on a regular basis to force the muscle to continue to adapt and change – that's where you begin to see the results of all your hard work!

The Seasons of Change

One of the main goals of a group instructor is to make sure they are changing up the workout on a regular basis for their classes. The instructor may or may not be thinking about what your individual physique goals might be. And that's something that's important for you to know before you go into classes –

Group classes are designed for *groups:* twenty – thirty people who may or may not have the same goals as you.

If your goal is weight loss, then you need to be doing the things that lead to weight loss, and that includes weight training and some cardio and eating right. However, if you are much further along as an athlete, your objectives may be different. For example, after I had lost all of my baby weight, my new goal was to build more muscle and more tone.

At that point I knew which muscle groups I needed to focus on more, and so I actually went to my group class instructor and said, here are some of my goals – *would you mind fitting this into one or two of our group classes?* She was happy to do so!

The end result was that I made that hour work for me, and as a side benefit, many others in the class became better acquainted with how to select weights for certain body parts.

A few weeks later we rotated in someone else's goals, and doing that became a fun thing for our class. We never knew who had requested what, but we knew someone in the class had asked for it and were open to trying it.

Seasonal Cycles at Fitness Clubs

This is something interesting you'll notice: gym class schedules are designed to fit into ninety-day intervals or two- or three-month sets before the gym changes them up. And here's why: athletic facilities work around their business cycles, just like any other company or business. They might do this to reflect natural cycles in their membership base or seasonal fluctuations – whether it's back to school, or get in shape season, or major summer break. As an example, gyms beef up their classes and make their schedules more robust at the beginning of the year to reflect the desire of all of those Americans who made New Years' resolutions to get in shape. You'll notice these cycles in the gyms and facilities that you work out in – and it will hold true regardless of the type of gym you attend, whether it's a hardcore, elite athletic facility, like CrossFit, or a more family-oriented fitness club.

The reason why this is beneficial to know is because it can be helpful to set a new fitness goal around the gym's business schedule. They often offer great deals on new memberships, personal training sessions, or other promotions at the beginning of the year, summer or for back-to-school, which can help to motivate you further. If you can use their schedule to help you attain the goal and get a great promotional deal on top of it, all the better!

When You Reach Your Goal, Set Another Goal!

Once you've reached your first goal, then challenge yourself to set and reach the next goal. The more you attend group classes or do this program, the stronger your body will become.

Perhaps you couldn't do a push-up on your toes when you first started training, but you can now do twenty in a row! Celebrate your success, but then immediately set another goal for yourself. For example, my next goal was to get into bikini competition shape. I didn't want to go on stage, I didn't care about competing and I didn't care about a trophy, but I knew I was getting ready for this book and needed to be in the best shape possible to be a great example so you would believe the information presented here is true.

That meant my body fat needed to be under 12 percent. But your next goal doesn't have to be anything like that – it might be to simply get back into your favorite pair of jeans. Whatever your goal is, the workouts I present here will help you achieve it.

The Scale Is a Big "FAT" Liar!

Remember what I said earlier, "The scale is a big "FAT" liar?" It's true! As you might remember, I said earlier that although I went from 26 percent body fat to 14 percent in about sixteen weeks, **my weight on the scale changed by only five pounds.** I want to repeat this here, in order to point out how vitally important it is that you use a more accurate way of measuring your progress, such as a tape measure or getting your body fat measured by a trained fitness professional who is knowledgeable about using body fat calipers.

If I had simply used the scale as an indicator, I would have gone weeks without knowing what my true progress was, other than how I looked in the mirror and felt in my clothes!

As women, we are far too dependent on the number
on that dial, no matter what else is changing about
our bodies. The danger is that especially when you're
new at this, it's far too likely that you'll think you're
making no progress, and that could dishearten
and discourage you. Don't trust that scale – it lies!

Recovery

Remember to let your body rest and recover. It's more important to stay on track with the food every day than it is to spend hours at a time in the gym. In fact, as I mentioned earlier, spending too much time working out can actually impede your progress, not propel it forward.

Warm up at the beginning of your training sessions to get your blood circulating, which will help your muscles fill up with fluid, get your heart rate going and increase your elasticity and flexibility. You can do some minimal stretching at the beginning, but the warm-up is more important. Stretching is more important at the *end* of the workout (more on that in a minute).

Lastly, build rest into your workout between sets and new exercises. Your rest time should be about one minute between sets and about three to five minutes between new exercises.

Drill this into your head: Recovery time, recovery time, recovery time! I see people in the gym all the time who spend two to three hours working out in back-to-back classes thinking it's helping them, because more should be better, right? Wrong. In reality they're just tearing down their bodies and immune systems because they are not giving themselves adequate time to recover and make changes.

So, here's a recap:

Remember, your muscle grows during its recovery state. When you're doing your workout, you're tearing the muscle down, but it's as it repairs itself that it begins to grow and activate. It can't build back up if you never give it enough recovery time.

Two Days On, One Day Off

The program I've personally had success with – reducing my risk of injury and keeping me at it consistently – is a two-day on, one-day off program. And remember you can have one cheat *meal* a week (it's not a cheat *day*, ladies!), or even one cheat meal every two weeks to make sure you're mentally rewarding yourself for your progress and satisfying the physical food cravings.

Stretch

Make sure that you stretch after every workout.
That's very important. Sometimes I see people at
the gym who use the last five minutes of class to
put their weights away instead of using that time as
the instructor intended it – for stretching out.
They're skipping the most important part of the workout!

The instructor, especially if they're good, designed
the stretching portion of the routine for the specific
muscles and muscle groups you've just worked.
There are particular stretches that you can do to help
those muscles recover quicker. It also helps to delay the
soreness you may have the next day. So please do yourself
a favor and stretch.

You surely don't want to risk getting injured needlessly, not when you'd still have
to take care of your baby while trying to recover! That's no fun at all, and you'd
just have weakened yourself at a time when your baby still needs you to be at 100
percent.

More Fit Mom Tips to Help Get You Started

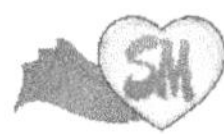

Cut out photos of your ideal physique so you have a concrete, realistic goal in your mind to achieve (can be of yourself, pre-pregnancy, or someone who has a similar build and a body you would like to have). Read motivational stories of others' transformations to keep you focused and on track.

Decide what your reward will be when you reach your goal, so you have something to aim for. For example, my reward was to buy a designer pair of gray skinny jeans with zippers at the ankles. I would envision going out in my new clothes and fit figure, and it motivated me to keep going.

To ease back into exercise after having a baby, begin with walking with your baby properly bundled and secured in a stroller as soon as your doctor gives you clearance. You will love this time together and the walking helps to kick-start your metabolism again. If your kids are older, you simply need the green light from your doctor and you can begin!

When your child naps, put in a 30-minute exercise video or do some quick at-home exercises to regain your muscle definition, coordination and energy. Again, you can join my Super Mom Get Fit Program and try it risk-free for 30 days at this link: *www.FitMomSecrets.com/Book-Offer*.

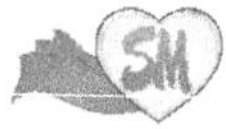

Find a gym that has good childcare so you can bring your baby during his Playtime (see Secrets of the Super Mom, Part I). It can be helpful to attend exercise classes in the early weeks after having a baby.

As we get older, estrogen levels fluctuate and we lose bone density, which predisposes us to osteoporosis and osteoarthritis. Resistance training and a high protein diet help keep our bones strong. Remember this: *"If your purse or child are heavier than the weights you use in the gym, then you won't make any changes!"* Don't be afraid to go heavy.

SECTION THREE
GETTING BACK INTO SUPER SHAPE

Margo Rodriguez, nutritionist and super mom of two boys says,

"Nursing helped me get back to my pre-baby shape, and it also helped that I am a nutritionist. I fully believe that 80 percent of what gets you back into great shape is the quality of your foods, eating a correct balance of foods, and eating small, frequent meals. I found it difficult to find time to work out after having a baby, so I focused all of my energy on healthy foods in the beginning. While I was home on maternity leave, I would DVR my favorite workouts on FIT TV – that was easiest for me so I could work out any time of the day."

Kelley Hendrickson, HR director and super mom of two girls says,

"I breastfed and that helped me get back into shape. I was lazy and didn't work out, which I'm now regretting. But I watched my food portions and got below my pre-baby weight."

Six-Week Post-Baby Workout

You can begin this workout as soon as you get your doctor's clearance that it's OK to exercise. If you had a vaginal delivery you can probably start within a week or two of having your baby, but if you had a c-section, your doctor will likely tell you to wait up to twelve weeks. Show your doctor this plan and communicate the exercises you want to start doing to make sure you get an official green light. Remember, if you've had any muscular injuries you may need to modify some of the higher risk exercises as noted. Video demonstrations are available through the Super Mom Get Fit Program at: *www.FitMomSecrets.com/Book-Offer.*

Mommy and Me Exercises

Peek-a-boo Squats (Newborn and up)

Place your baby in his stroller or high chair. Either cover your eyes or your baby's eyes with your hands and squat down, keeping your knees above your toes and squatting no more than ninety degrees from the floor. Inhale as you squat down, exhale as you come up, and say, "Peek-a-boo!" as you uncover your eyes. This is a great exercise for your quadriceps and glutes. Make sure to squeeze your bottom tight as you rise up. You can even use a stroller blanket or cloth diaper to cover your baby's face as you do the "Peek-a-boo!" to make it more fun. **Do twelve – fifteen reps for three sets.**

Baby-Back Walking Lunges (Newborn and up)

This is another great legs and glutes workout. Use a Baby Bjorn or secure baby wrap to attach your baby to your chest or back, depending on the age of the child. Do walking lunges in your home, alternating legs, so you get a great workout while your baby gets a fun ride around the house! Again, inhale as you come down, pause and exhale as you come up. Alternate legs, and try to get a deep lunge, but make sure to always maintain a ninety-degree angle or more. **Do twelve – fifteen reps for three sets.**

Rock and Rolls (Six months and up, or until child has good head stability)

Luke and I often do this one together in gymnastics. Sit on the floor in a pike position and put your baby on your lap, facing away from you. Next, wrap your arms around his legs and pull him into a tuck position. Roll backward and up again, working your abdominals. This is a good workout for your abs while you teach your baby how to tuck and roll – and it's a blast for your child!

Forward Rolls (Twelve - fifteen months and up)

This is another gymnastics move, but it took me some time to master it, as I was always worried I would hurt his neck. There are two versions to this one.

1. Your child faces away from you and you are on your knees as you spot him. Secure his hips straight with your arm and have him place his hands on the floor as he bends over.

Then, tuck his head into his chest as you help him do a forward roll with your other arm, continually spotting him with your original arm in set position as you bring his hips up and over.

2. Another version is to do a forward roll as your child watches and then help him do one. It helps if you have a cushy yoga mat on the floor to help him learn how to roll over. Again, you'll need to support his head and neck and make sure he tucks it in tightly to his chest. Spot him with your arms to help him roll over straight and not fall sideways.

Roll-Overs (Six months and up)

This was a fun, silly exercise I did with Luke when I wanted to teach him how to roll over on his own both ways. First, put your baby on his tummy or Bumbo seat so he can watch you. Lie on the floor and put your arms above your head. Pull in your tummy and tighten your glutes, and then lead with one of your shoulders to roll all the way over. Sing the song, "Ten in the Bed" (or as I call it, the "Roll Over" song!) as you do this so your child learns that this is what you're doing. Next, help your baby do the same thing you just did, singing the "Roll Over" song as you go. **Do twelve – fifteen reps for three sets.**

Ball Squeeze and Toss (Six months and up)

Get a lightweight plastic ball about eight inches in diameter. Sit with the ball in between your knees on top of your workout bench. Do three squeezes of your inner thighs and count excitedly to your child, "One, two, three!" On the count of three, lightly toss the ball to your child and ask him to toss it back. He might not know how to do this yet, but he'll still enjoy the game. This is a fun way to play catch and work out your inner thighs at the same time. **Do twelve – fifteen reps for three sets.**

Balance Beam Walk / Backward Squats (Twelve months and up or when walking well)

With painter's or masking tape, mark out a faux balance beam on the floor, about eight feet long and six inches wide. Take your toddler's hands and let him face you while you squat in front of him. The object is for your toddler to walk on the "beam" while you perform backward pulse squats. Once you're at the end of the beam, turn around and do it again. You can even teach your child how to walk backwards with this move, which is really fun for them. **Do twelve – fifteen reps for three sets.**

Pony Ride Leg Extensions (Nine months and up)

Sit down on a chair and place your baby or toddler on your ankles while facing you. Hold his hands securely and slowly bring your feet up almost to the top, but keep a slight bend in your knees. Bring him down again slowly – inhale as you bring him up, exhale as you go down to mimic a leg extension exercise. Sing songs and be silly, but keep your form in mind. **Do twelve – fifteen reps for three set**s.

> ➡ Option 2: Move your child to your lap and keep your toes planted on the floor while raising your heels up and down. This is a seated calf raise. You can also turn your toes in on one set and out on another to work your calves at different angles.

Baby Bridges (Six months and up)

Lie on your back with your knees bent and feet flat on the floor in front of you. Place your baby facing you on top of your lower abdomen. Bring your hips up off the floor and squeeze your glutes tightly. **Do twelve – fifteen reps for three sets.**

Push-up Kisses (Newborn and up)

Place your baby face-up on a soft blanket on the floor. Get into push-up position, either on your knees or toes (whatever you are able to do) over your baby, keeping all your weight above your shoulders and chest. As you come down to perform your push-up, give your little one a kiss before pushing yourself back up again. Inhale as you come down and exhale as you come up. Do any many as you can in sets of twenty. Work up to doing push-ups on your toes, but you can still get a great chest and back workout on your knees.

Side Plank Wraps (Newborn and up)

This is a slight variation on the Push-up Kisses exercise. Again, place your baby face-up on a soft blanket on the floor. Instead of push-up position, though, you get into a side-plank position with your elbow on the floor in alignment with your shoulder and feet extended, hips lifted. Come in to do a twist with your elevated arm, give your baby a kiss and come back up, resuming the side-plank position.

This is an advanced move and it might take some time to build the necessary upper body strength. **Start with three sets of five – eight reps and increase them as you become stronger.**

Super Tummy Time (Newborn and up)

Physicians recommend infants get adequate Tummy Time daily to build up their head and upper body strength. Well, it only makes sense for you to do a Tummy Time workout with your baby! While he's enjoying his Tummy Time, you also get on your tummy and do a series of "Supermans," er, "Super Moms!" Tighten your abdomen as you lift both of your arms and legs, squeezing your glutes.

Make sure to keep your head and neck neutral, but make silly faces and noises to your baby who is probably thrilled to have a workout buddy! Next, stretch out your right arm and your left leg, then switch to the left arm and right leg to increase your balance and stability. **Repeat twelve – fifteen reps for three sets.**

Baby Biceps (Three - four months and up)

Hold your baby under his arms in front of you with both hands. Lift him up while keeping the tension on the muscle the entire time. Inhale as you bring him up, exhale as you bring him down, but do not rest in between reps. Repeat eight – ten reps of as many sets as your baby enjoys.

You can switch grips by turning your palms in and holding your baby in the same place under his arms. Now the move becomes a simulated hammer curl. Make sure the grip is comfortable and safe for your baby.

Fun Front Raises (Three - four months and up)

Hold your baby under his arms in front of you with both hands, with your palms facing down. The slight change in the orientation of your hands turns the move into a shoulder exercise instead of biceps. Lift your baby up to the point where your arms are parallel to your shoulders, but no higher. The age of the child varies on this one, as I definitely recommend waiting until your baby has good head stability. Keep all movements slow and inhale as you bring him up, exhale as you lower him. **Repeat ten – twelve reps for three sets.**

Stroller-Walking Lunges (Newborn and up)

The very first exercise I began right after my babies were born was the stroller walk. There's nothing like the enjoyment and freedom you feel as you take your brand new little one out for a little walk and sunshine. The jogging stroller definitely helps you get in some good resistance because, even if you were a jogger before, you didn't have to push twenty-plus pounds in front of you at the same time!

Another great leg and glutes workout is to do stroller-walking lunges as you push your little one for his walk.

Use the stroller handles to help you keep your balance and do this move slowly, inhaling as you come down and exhaling as you rise back up again, careful not to over-extend your knees over your toes. Come down as far as you can on the lunge and try to get in a good deep stretch, up to a ninety-degree angle. Always push up with the leg in front. Switch legs and do as many as you can, but make sure to count so you know your starting point for the next time. **Do twelve - fifteen reps for three sets.**

Super Shoulder Presses (Around 4 - 5 months and up)

Similar to the Baby Biceps and Fun Front Raises: Lift your baby from under his arms, putting one of your feet back for support. Instead of keeping your baby in front of you the whole time, lift him higher like an incline chest or shoulder press. Bring him into you, give him a kiss, and bring him back out. **Repeat ten – twelve reps for three sets.**

Side Lateral Toy Tosses (Newborn and up)

Playtime's over and we need to pick up some toys! Tighten your abs and glutes as you stand in a wide squat stance. Bend your legs and bring your opposite arm to your opposite foot, pick up a toy that's near you and toss it into the toy box.

The important thing about this exercise (aside from getting rid of clutter!) is to keep your form. As you bend down to opposing sides, keep your chest and head lifted up. All the work is in the legs, abs and glutes, but not the back! Repeat ten – twelve reps for three sets or until all the toys are gone! Your child gets the joy of watching you work, but even though he's not doing much else during this one, he's still learning by example. Putting toys away must be cool if Mom's doing it, right?

Jumping Jacks / Plyos (Newborn and up)

Even if your baby can't do a jumping jack yet, you can still show him it's fun to be fit and active. Do this during your baby's Playtime (see *Secrets of the Super Moms, Part I*) as he lies or sits on a blanket with toys.

Pick any three and do fifteen reps for three sets of these exercises:

- Jumping Jacks
- High Knees
- Side-to-Side Jumps
- Skis
- Repeater Knees on each side

- Burpees (add a tuck jump at the end for an advanced move)
- High-low Punches

(Kickboxing)

- High-low Kicks
- Side Knee Kicks

Workout in a Box

It may surprise you when I tell you that you don't need to spend a ton of money or have an entire room in your house devoted to a home gym. With some very basic equipment, you can get the same results as, or better than going to the gym, and you can save the drive-time and fit it in around your baby's nap schedule by doing it at home.

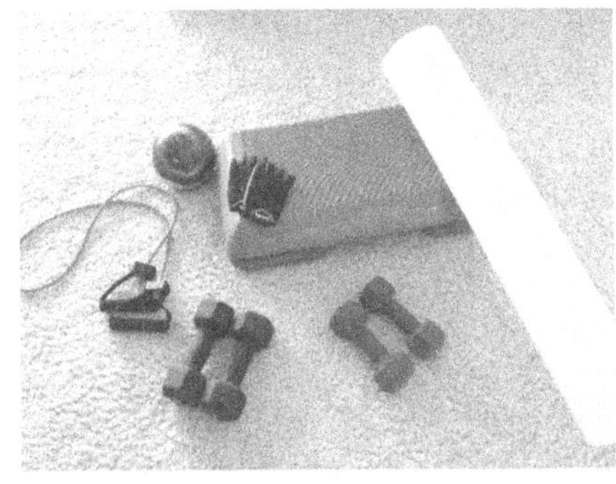

I understand how difficult it can be to fit in precious exercise time around a baby's routine. There have been days when I've had to pre-plan and make meals the day before, wake up thirty minutes earlier or pack what feels like the entire baby's room, just to make it to the gym and put even more stress on my body. (*What are we, CRAZY?!*) So here are some tips you can use to get the job done just as effectively and save a little extra time.

Equipment

All you need to get started are:

- **Three sets of dumbbells** (5 lb, 8 lb and 10 lb) – For a full set of three, it will cost around $27.

- **Step bench with two risers** on each side – Costs about $30.

- **Exercise mat** – Costs about $13.

- **Resistance bands** – A set of three, small, medium and large resistance, costs $10.50.

- **Eight-inch weighted ball** (6 – 8 lb) – About $19.

- **Pair of resistance training gloves** – About $15.

- **Foam roller** – About $14.

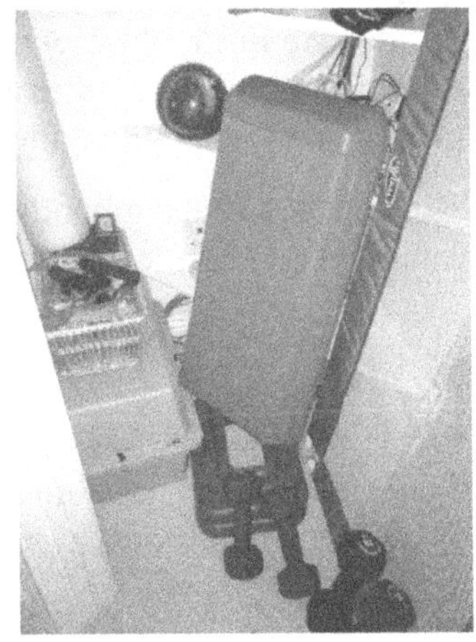

The bonus of a small kit like this one is all your equipment can fit into a small closet or under a bed for easy storage. And with these tools, you can get a complete "home gym" for less than $130.

Dumbbells

When I first started training, I had to use 5 lb weights for arms and shoulders. I should say here that although legs, back and glutes are larger muscles and they can take more weight, when I first started out I would only do 8 – 10 lbs on those, too.

It's OK, and even smart, to start slow, but increase your resistance as you feel your body getting stronger. Remember, the last three reps of your set should be difficult, but not impossible. If you're having to engage other muscles than the ones you're working to complete an exercise, then the weight is too heavy and you need to drop down.

The benefit of having a set of three, like I'm recommending, is to work different muscle groups according to their strength level.

Bench with Risers

Even if you're not into the latest Step moves, getting a bench with risers is a great way to do chest presses, one-arm rows and push-ups until you're strong enough to do them on the floor, plus a whole list of other important exercises. Additionally, when you do bench dips, as recommended in the Advanced Workout, you'll be able to get the full range of motion on the exercise without bouncing your bottom up and down on the floor. I like this tool for certain exercises like chest presses, because you can pull your shoulders to the point where they are level with the bench (no lower to protect them from injury) without having to stop at the floor.

The bench is also a great tool to use to assist you with completing exercises you cannot yet do on the floor, such as lat push-ups or mountain climbers.

Exercise Mat

You need this for stretching and to put on your bench and give yourself a little cushion whenever you perform moves where you have to lie on top of the bench on your back.

Resistance Bands

Resistance bands are a great counterpoint to using dumbbells because they focus the tension on the muscles differently. You hold them differently and work the angles of the exercise differently with bands than you do with dumbbells.

This is a great, inexpensive way to work the exact same exercise as you would with a dumbbell, but "trick" your body into thinking it's doing something completely different. And the benefit of that: quicker results!

Weighted Ball

When you do abdominal exercises, adding a weighted ball to the mix is a great way to increase your challenge and get more variety. It's a terrific addition to your Workout in a Box.

Resistance Gloves

You can certainly do all your exercises without workout gloves, but I like them because they protect the insides of my hands from getting calluses, which often split. Plus, who wouldn't feel like a badass Super Mom with cool resistance gloves?

I definitely believe new workout gear, such as a new top or fitted workout pants can motivate you to perform. You still don't have to spend a lot of money to achieve this, but the gloves empower you AND they are practical for your hands.

Foam Roller

If you're new to working out, you might be surprised to see how absolutely sore your body gets! You may even wonder, *"Why am I even doing this? I can't even walk today!"* But I'm here to tell you it will get better as you get stronger, and there are lots of things you can do to relieve soreness. One of them is stretching and massaging tired muscle groups with this foam roller. You can roll whatever body part is in pain or in need of massaging and you choose the amount of pressure. This foam roller can save you many trips to the massage therapist, and it's cheap!

Post-Delivery 6-Week Workout

Remember to rest about one minute in between sets, as long as it takes for your breathing to return to normal. The break in between exercises should be around three to five minutes, or as long as it takes to get your baby or child set up for the next one.

As a warm-up, you can do ten minutes of stroller walking or one set of each of these exercises. Make sure you have your doctor's clearance before beginning, take your time and remember; you're doing this for yourself as well as for your baby. This program assumes you're beginning these exercises after a minimum of twelve weeks recovery time if you've had a c-section.

Week 1 - New Beginnings

Although we've already talked about how to break up the muscle groups and why, when you start the first week of this program I don't have specific muscle groups listed, and the reason for that is because your goal for the first week is simply to get some movement and a little cardio for your heart. If you've been inactive for your entire pregnancy, it's very important to ease back into activity. Take your time, catch your breath, enjoy the time with your baby. Those are your only goals for the first couple of weeks.

As you begin to feel stronger and have more energy, then you can proceed to the other muscle groups, but again, proceed with caution and only with your doctor's permission! Make sure to stretch at the end of every workout. *For all exercises, perform 3 sets of each, and 12 - 15 reps per set, unless otherwise noted.*

Day of the Week		Exercises
Monday		Stroller walk for 30 minutes; stretch
Tuesday		Stroller walk for 30 minutes; stretch
Wednesday	Rest	Play outside for 15 minutes
Thursday		Rest
Friday		Power stroller walk for 35 minutes; 3 sets of Stroller-Walking Lunges
Saturday		Stroller walk for 10 minutes for warm-up
		3 sets of Stroller-Walking Lunges
		3 sets of Baby Back Walking Lunges
		3 sets of Peek-a-Boo squats
Sunday	Rest	Play outside for 15 minutes

Week 2 - Muscle Engagement

Day of the Week		Exercises
Monday	Back and Biceps	Stroller walk for 15 minutes for warm-up
		3 sets of Baby Biceps
		3 sets of Baby Hammer Curls
		3 sets of Push-up Kisses
		1 set of Side Lateral Toy Tosses
Tuesday	Fat Burning	Stroller walk for 30 minutes; stretch
Wednesday	Legs and Glutes	Stroller walk for 15 minutes for warm-up
		1 set of Stroller-Walking Lunges
		3 sets of Wide Grip Push-up Kisses
		3 sets of Fun Front Raises
		3 sets of Super Shoulder Presses
Thursday	Rest	
Friday	Abs and Glutes	Power stroller walk for 15 minutes
		3 sets of Roll-overs
		3 sets of Super Tummy Time
		3 sets of Baby Back Walking Lunges
		3 sets of Baby Bridges
Saturday	Chest and Shoulders	Stroller walk for 10 minutes for warm-up
		3 sets of Ball Squeeze and Tosses
		3 sets of Super Shoulder Presses
		3 sets of Push-up Kisses
		2 sets of Side Plank Wraps
Sunday	Rest	Play outside for 15 minutes

Week 3 - Muscle Activation

Day of the Week		Exercises
Monday	Chest, Shoulders and Triceps	Power stroller walk for 15 minutes; stretch
		Push-up Kisses
		Side Plank Wraps
		Super Presses
		Jumping Jacks / Plyos
Tuesday	Back and Biceps	Stroller walk for 30 minutes; stretch
		Baby Biceps
		Baby Hammer Curls
		Rock and Rolls
		Roll-overs
Wednesday	Rest	Stroller walk for 30 minutes; stretch
Thursday	Legs	Peek-a-Boo Squats
		Backward Squats (Balance beam)
		Pony Ride Leg Extensions
		Side Lateral Toy Tosses
Friday	Fat Burning	Power stroller walk for 35 minutes; 3 sets of Stroller-Walking Lunges
Saturday	Chest, Shoulders and Triceps	Push-up Kisses
		Side Plank Wraps
		Super Tummy Time
		Jumping Jacks / Plyos
Sunday	Rest	Play outside for 30 minutes

Week 4 - Muscle Activation

Day of the Week		Exercises
Monday	Legs	Power stroller walk for 15 minutes; stretch
		Stroller-Walking Lunges
		Baby Bridges
		Ball Squeeze and Tosses
		Baby Back Walking Lunges
Tuesday	Back and Biceps	Stroller walk for 20 minutes; stretch
		Baby Biceps
		Baby Hammer Curls
		Wide-grip Push-up Kisses
Wednesday	Rest	Stroller walk for 30 minutes; stretch
Thursday	Chest, Shoulders and Triceps	Super Shoulder Presses
		Side Plank Wraps
		Super Tummy Time
		Side Lateral Toy Tosses
Friday	Fat Burning	Power stroller walk for 35 minutes; 3 sets of Stroller-Walking Lunges
Saturday	Legs	Baby Back Alternating Walking Lunges
		Peek-a-Boo Squats
		Pony Ride Leg Extensions
		Stroller-Walking Lunges
Sunday	Rest	Play outside for 30 minutes

Week 5 - Muscle Endurance

Day of the Week		Exercises
Monday	Back and Biceps	Power stroller walk for 15 minutes; stretch
		Baby Biceps
		Baby Hammer Curls
		Wide Push-up Kisses
Tuesday	Chest, Shoulders and Triceps	Super Shoulder Presses
		Fun Front Raises
		Side Plank Wraps
		Super Tummy Time
		Side Lateral Toy Tosses
Wednesday	Rest	Stroller walk for 30 minutes; stretch
Thursday	Legs	Power stroller walk for 15 minutes; stretch
		Stroller-Walking Lunges
		Baby Bridges
		Ball Squeeze and Tosses
		Baby Back Walking Lunges
Friday	Fat Burning	Power stroller walk for 35 minutes; 3 sets of Stroller-Walking Lunges
Saturday	Back and Biceps	Wide Push-up Kisses
		Baby Biceps
		Baby Hammer Curls
		Jumping Jacks / Plyos
Sunday	Rest	Play outside for 30 minutes

Week 6 - Muscle Endurance

Day of the Week		Exercises
Monday	Legs	Power stroller walk for 15 minutes; stretch
		Baby Back Walking Lunges
		Baby Back Alternating Walking Lunges
		Peek-a-Boo Squats
		Pony Ride Leg Extensions
		Stroller-Walking Lunges
Tuesday	Back and Biceps	Stroller walk for 20 minutes; stretch
		Baby Biceps
		Baby Hammer Curls
		Wide-grip Push-up Kisses
Wednesday	Rest	Stroller walk for 30 minutes; stretch
Thursday	Chest, Shoulders and Triceps	Super Shoulder Presses
		Side Plank Wraps
		Super Tummy Time
		Side Lateral Toy Tosses
Friday	Fat Burning	Power stroller walk for 35 minutes; 3 sets of Stroller-Walking Lunges
Saturday	Legs	Power stroller walk for 15 minutes; stretch
		Stroller-Walking Lunges
		Baby Bridges
		Ball Squeeze and Tosses
Sunday	Rest	Play outside for 30 minutes

The Exercises

BACK

Bent-over Dumbbell Row

Hold a dumbbell in each hand. While keeping your knees slightly bent, tip forward from the hip, keeping your chest and head up. Keep your back straight as you pull your shoulder blades straight back. Your elbows should go up toward the ceiling, not out to the side. Inhale as you pull the weights up. Exhale and lower them slowly to knee level. As you move your arms back to the starting position, be careful not to roll your shoulders.

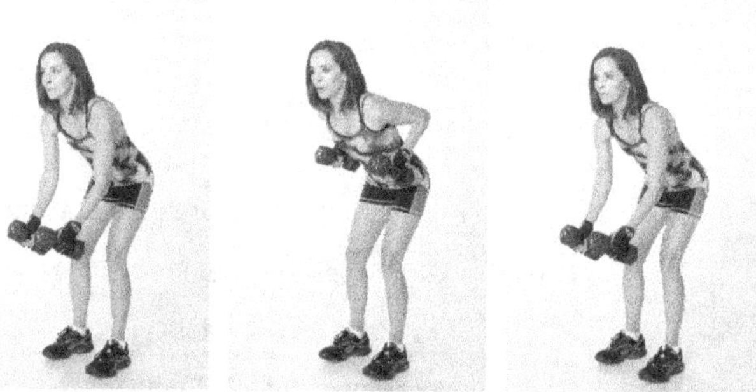

One-Arm Dumbbell Row

Set up a bench with one or two risers for stability. Place one foot up on the bench as you stabilize yourself in a forward lunge. Bend over and rest the arm on the same side as your lunging leg on that leg as you lift a dumbbell with the other arm. Pull your elbow straight back toward the ceiling, keeping your elbow close to your body. Inhale as you pull the dumbbell up. Exhale and lower it slowly to the set position, which is just opposite the other (bent) leg.

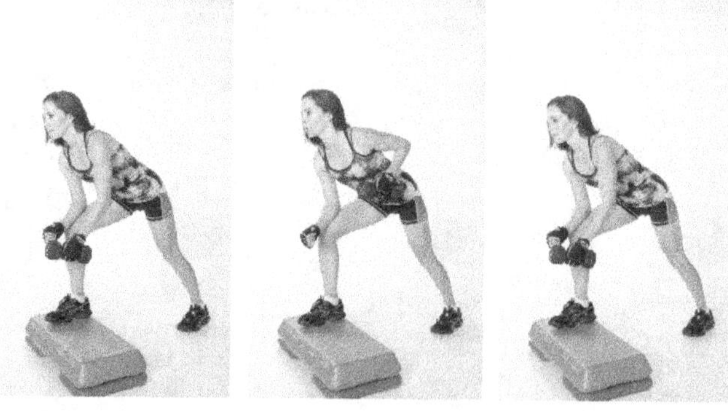

Reverse-Grip Dumbbell Row

Stand with your feet about shoulder-width apart and a heavy dumbbell in each hand, palms facing out. Bend over slightly and keep your legs slightly bent.

Inhale and squeeze your shoulder blades together while keeping your arms close to your body and pointing your elbows straight back. Keep your head and chest up. Exhale and lower the weights to about knee level.

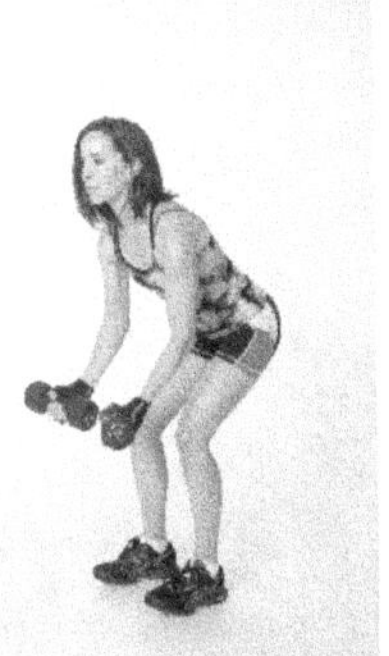 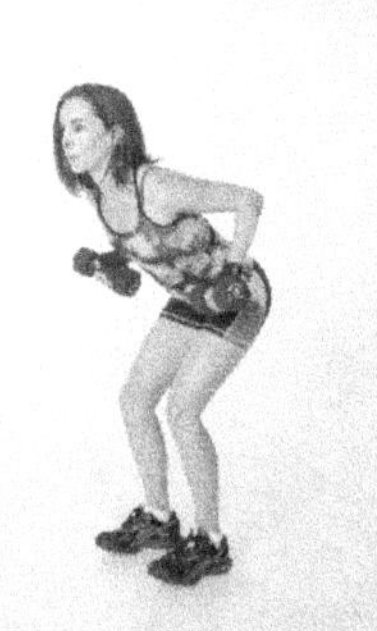 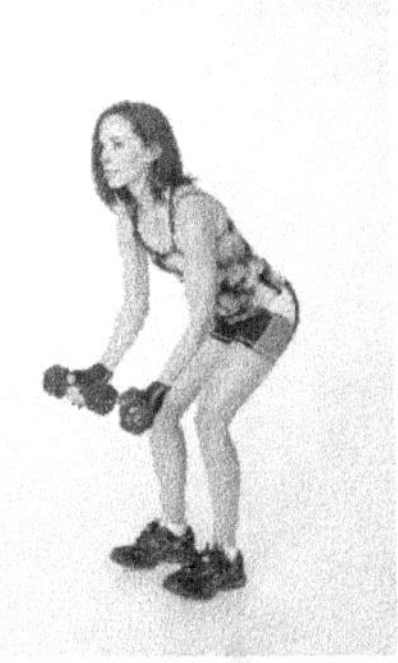

Band Pull-downs

> ### FIT MOM TIP:
>
> This is a back exercise, so make sure to squeeze the back muscles as you pull the band down. Otherwise, you'll work the shoulders and biceps and forfeit the back exercise altogether.

Stand with a medium to heavy resistance band. Loop your hands inside the handles and then hold the band firmly with both hands. Start with your arms outstretched over your head. Exhale as you pull the band apart and down behind your head, stopping when your arms are bent at 90-degree angles at the elbow. Inhale as you slowly release the band back to the starting position.

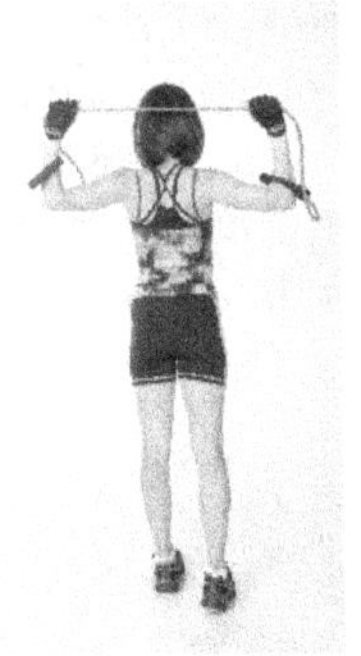 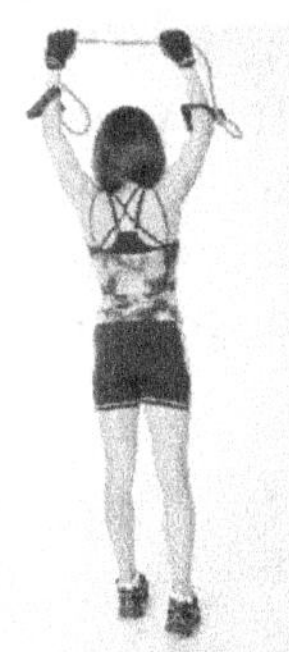 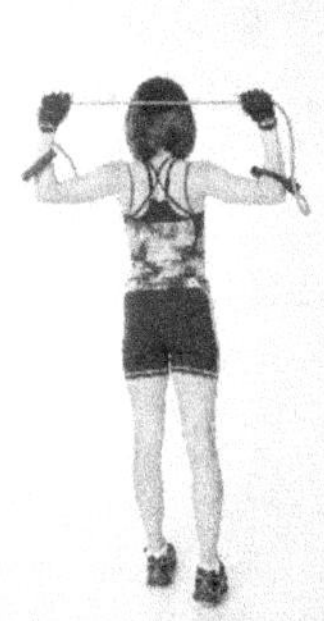

Dumbbell Deadlift

Stand with your feet about shoulder-width apart and hold a heavy dumbbell in each hand (typically 12- or 15-pound dumbbells). Bend forward at the waist, keeping the dumbbells close to your body, and inhale as you keep your back straight while lowering the weights to knee level. Exhale as you stand up, forcing the weight into the backs of your heels. Keep your back straight and knees slightly bent the entire time.

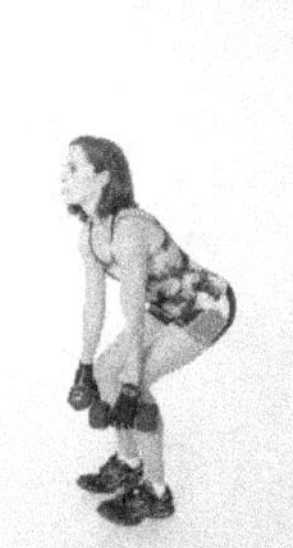 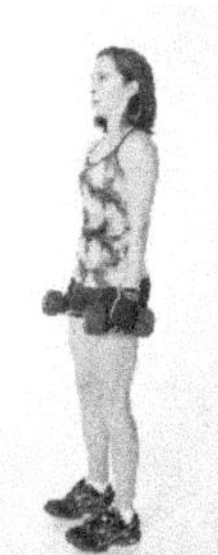 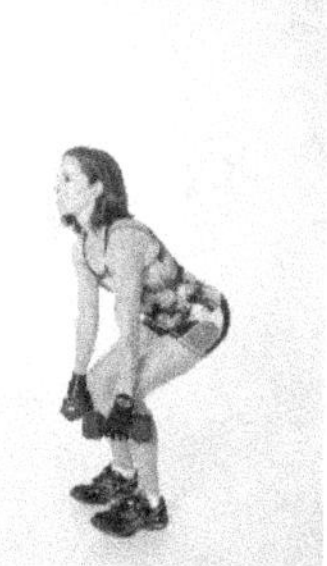

ARMS

Standing Dumbbell Curl

For a traditional standing dumbbell curl, you want your feet to be shoulder-width apart, feet facing forward and knees slightly bent. You can also stand in what is called a "split stance," where you have one foot back on the ball of your foot for support. Sometimes I'll do the split stance if I'm going a little heavier on the weights to relieve my lower back from trying to take on the load for my arms. Palms face out, and you keep your arms close to your body the entire time. Exhale as you bring the dumbbells up to your shoulder. Turn your arms slightly in at the top of the move to focus more on the bicep muscle. This slight twist at the top helps to put a nice curved peak on your bicep. Inhale as you keep the tension on the muscle and come down to the starting position. Make sure to keep the tempo relatively consistent as you do the curls.

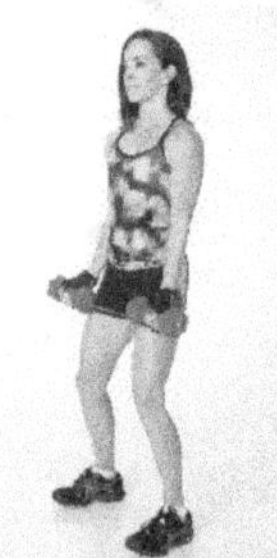 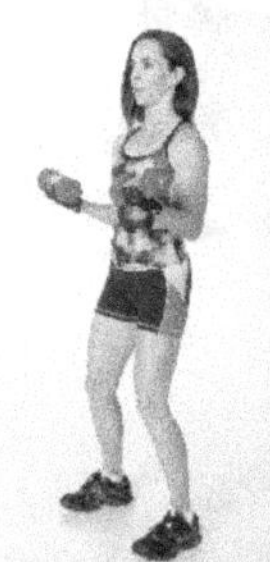 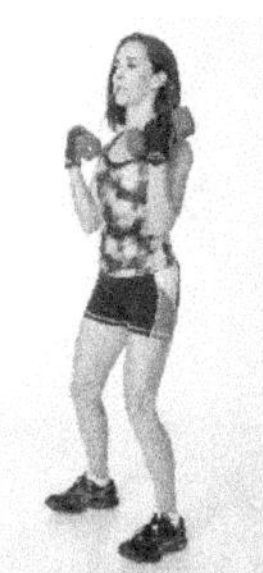

Standing Hammer Dumbbell Curl

You can do hammer curls either standing or seated. To do them standing, start in the same position as you did for the standing dumbbell curl, but instead of palms facing out, they face each other (inward to your body).

Inhale and curl the dumbbells alternately, bringing one up as you bring the other down. Exhale as you bring them down. Keep the end of the dumbbell facing up toward the ceiling the entire time – when in motion, it gives the appearance that you're holding a hammer.

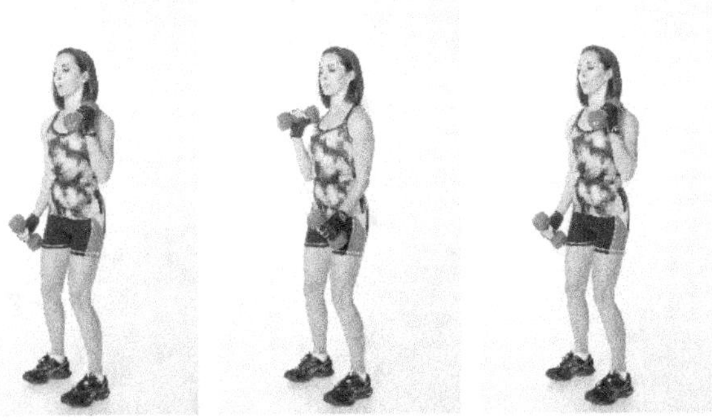

Extended Biceps Curl

As with the traditional Standing Biceps Curl, palms face out for this exercise. But instead of keeping your arms close, you keep your elbows close, but extend your forearms out with your palms facing up. Exhale as you bring the dumbbells up to your shoulder. Inhale as you bring your arms back down as far as they can comfortably go and keep a slight bend in the elbow.

Make sure to keep the tempo relatively consistent as you do the curls.

FIT MOM TIP:

To protect your back and make sure you stand properly for this exercise, you can put one foot up on the bench just for support.

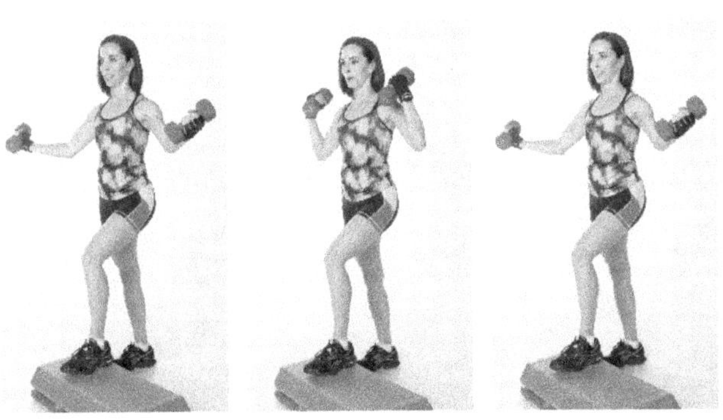

Concentration Curl

Sit on a workout bench or step, as shown here. Hold a dumbbell in your right hand, using your right inner thigh for support. (**Fit Mom Tip:** I like to use my elbow as a rough gauge for placement, but you want to keep your legs strongly in place and prevent your lifting arm from slipping.) Inhale as you bring the dumbbell in an arc pattern across your body until the dumbbell reaches your shoulder. Pause at the top, squeezing the bicep muscle for emphasis. Exhale as you bring the dumbbell back to the starting position. After you complete a full set on the right bicep, switch to the left bicep and continue.

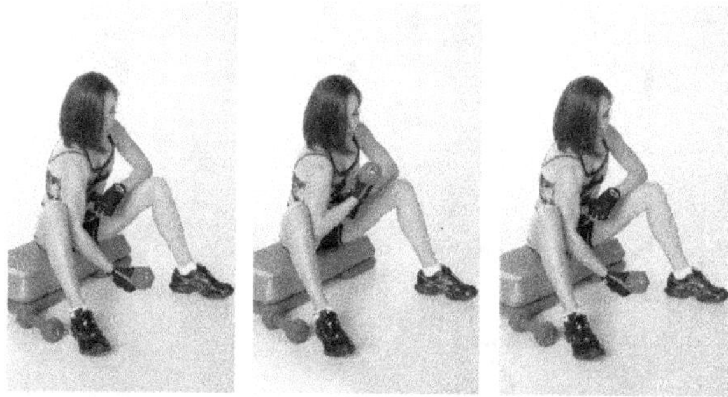

Reverse Lunge with Dumbbell Curl

This is a more advanced exercise, because it involves several movements in one. The most important thing is to maintain good form and balance the entire time. If you're not strong enough yet to do a compound movement like this one, it's best to simply do stationary lunges on the floor and leave out the curl.

Hold two dumbbells and step up on a bench, like this one. Step forward with one foot and get your placement set. Inhale as you lunge on the forward leg, keeping your body straight and dipping until your forward leg is parallel to the floor. Exhale as you return to position, pushing up with the heel of the forward foot and squeezing your glutes on the way up. Keep your knees slightly bent the entire time.

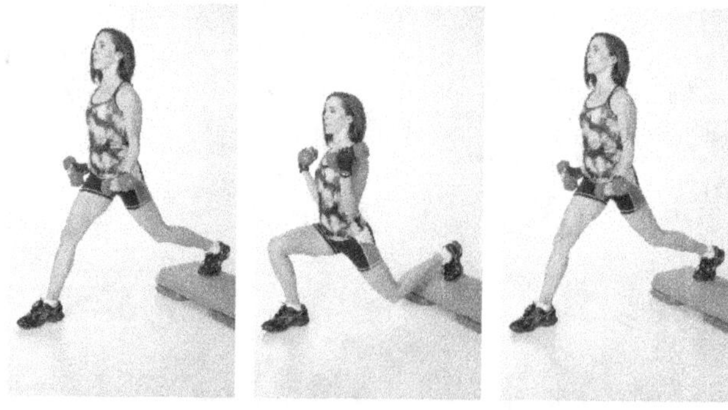

Biceps Curl with Bands

This exercise is similar to the Standing Dumbbell Curl, but it stimulates the muscle differently, using a different workout tool, such as the bands. Resistance bands vary in their strength. I use one of the more difficult ones – you can purchase a set of three at any sporting goods store for about $15. When doing this exercise, choose the moderate to difficult one. You can also make this exercise more difficult by placing both feet on top of the band, as shown. To reduce the difficulty, put only one foot on top of the band.

Place two feet on top of a band, about shoulder-width apart. Using the handles, curl the bands up to your shoulder, exhaling as you do so. Inhale as you bring your hands back down.

> **FIT MOM TIP:**
>
> To get a nice peak on the bicep, turn your pinkies in slightly toward your shoulders to get a nice little twist at the top.

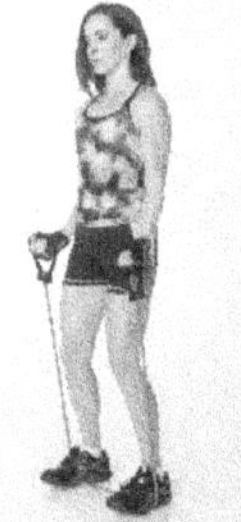 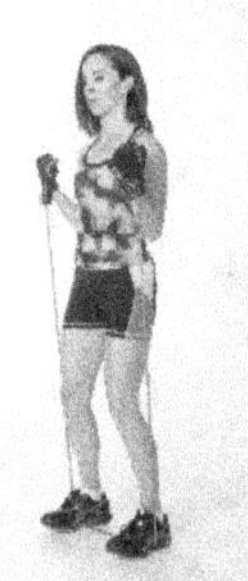 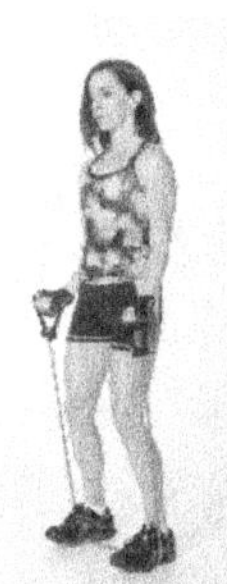

TRICEPS

Overhead Triceps Extension

You can do this exercise seated or standing, and it's good to alternate between the two to stress the muscle differently and get it to respond.

Grab one heavy dumbbell and lift it over your head, keeping your elbow in close to your ear and your palm facing out. Inhale as you slowly lower the dumbbell behind your head to the upper part of your back. Exhale as you return to the starting position.

Remember, good form for this exercise is keeping your arms close to your head with your elbows pointed toward the ceiling.

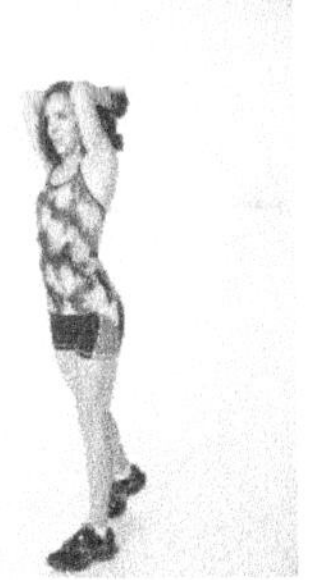 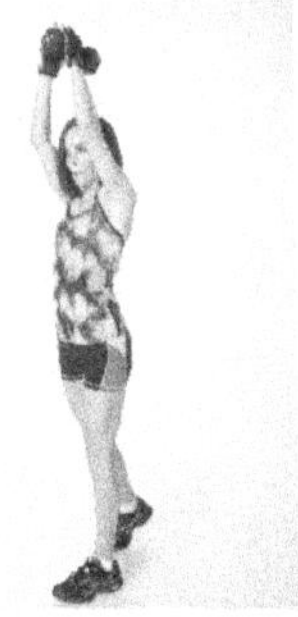

Bench Dips

Sit on the edge of a workout bench, either one from the gym or a step bench with risers as shown here. Place your palms straight down on the edge of the bench with your fingers facing forward and bring your feet out as far as you can and still hold up your body weight. Inhale as you lower your body until your upper arms are parallel to the floor. Exhale as you push up, locking your elbows. Keep your bottom close to the bench at all times. Otherwise, you're working the shoulders too hard and in a bad form position.

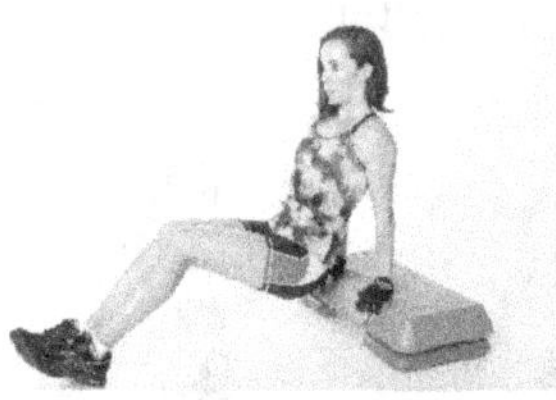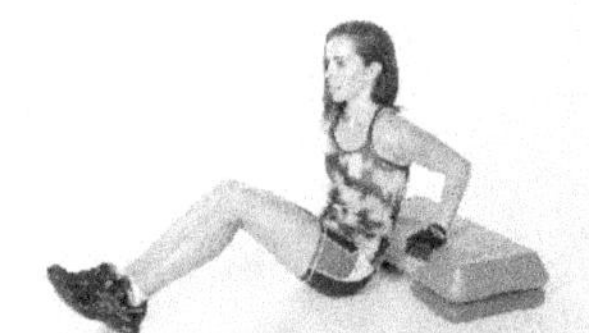

Triceps Pushups

This is a very difficult pushup because the focus is almost entirely on your small triceps muscles. If you do this on your toes, remember, you're doing it with your entire body weight! Impressive!

To begin this exercise, place your hands in a small triangle on the floor in front of you. Inhale as you come down until your chest is right above the floor, and exhale as you push up.

The secret to doing this exercise correctly is to keep your arms close to your body with your elbows pointed up toward the ceiling.

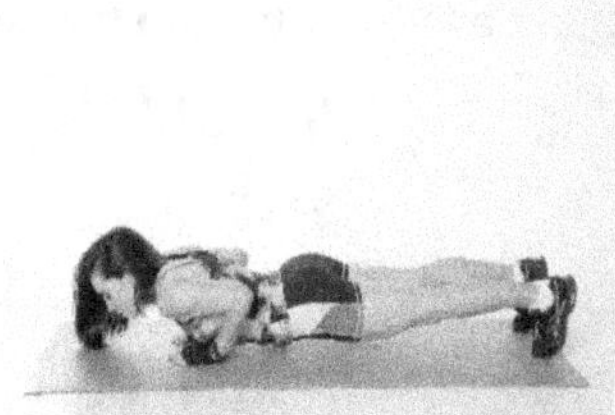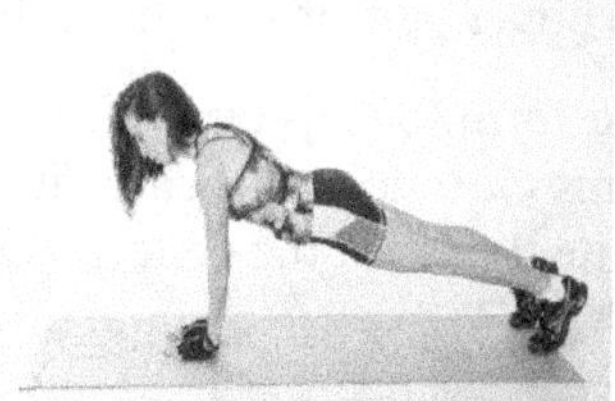

Triceps Kickbacks

Lean forward with one arm resting on one leg in a modified runner's lunge position. You can also do this exercise on a workout bench. Start with your lifting arm in a 90-degree angle.

Exhale as you use your triceps muscle to lift the weight until the arm is fully extended.

Pause at the top, inhale, and lower the dumbbell back to the starting position.

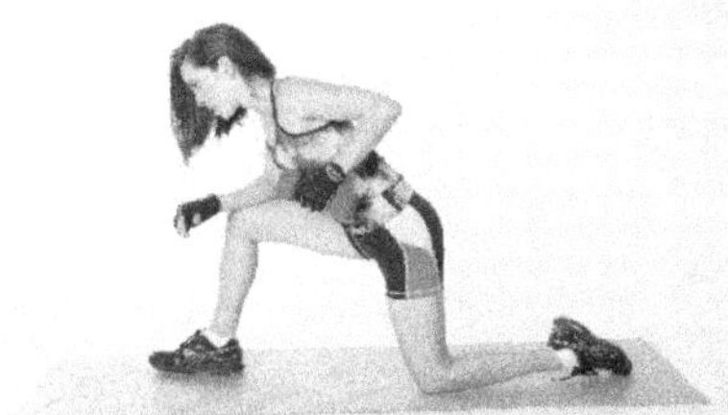 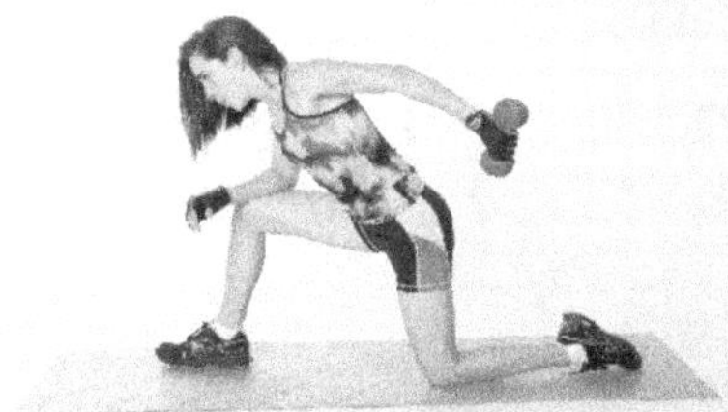

CHEST

Dumbbell Chest Press

You can do this exercise with a barbell – however, for at-home workouts, I prefer this style, which is safer, easier to control, and more practical for fitting in around a child's schedule.

Lie down on a soft mat placed on the top of your bench with two risers flat on the floor. (This image shows the correct positioning, but the bench has been adjusted for the incline position. You can do the exact same thing with the bench flat.) Your feet should lie flat on the floor. Hold a dumbbell in each hand just above your chest, with your palms facing your feet (keep your wrists straight and aligned with the elbow as you perform the move).

Inhale as you bring the weights down, bending your elbows and forming a ninety-degree angle. Exhale as you push the weights back up above your chest. Repeat the move and make sure to keep the weights aligned no lower than your shoulders in the inhale position.

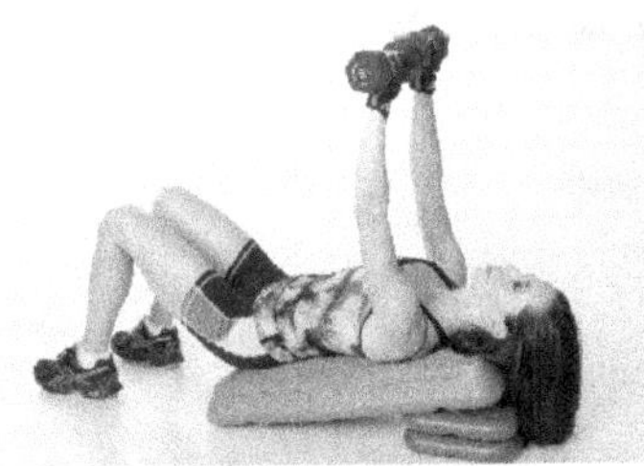 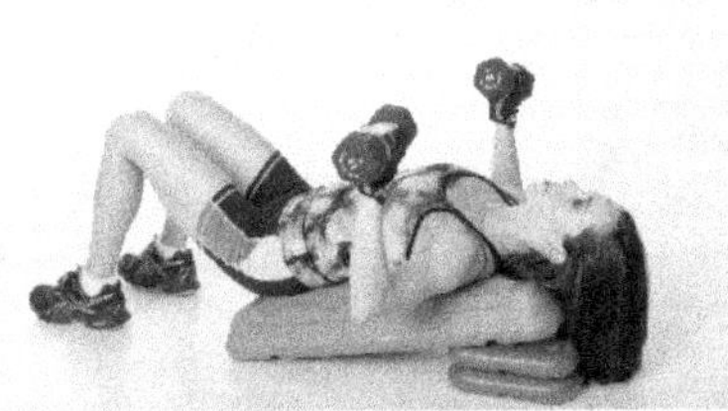

Incline Chest Press

You can do this exercise with a barbell or dumbbells, but I find I get a better range of motion with dumbbells without overstressing my forearms.

Lie down on a soft mat placed on the top of your bench positioned at an incline (as shown here). Your feet should lie flat on the floor. Hold a dumbbell in each hand just above your chest, with your palms facing your feet. Inhale as you bring the weights down, bending your elbows and forming a 90-degree angle until they are level with your shoulders.

Exhale as you push the weights back to the starting position. Keep a slight bend in the elbow the entire time.

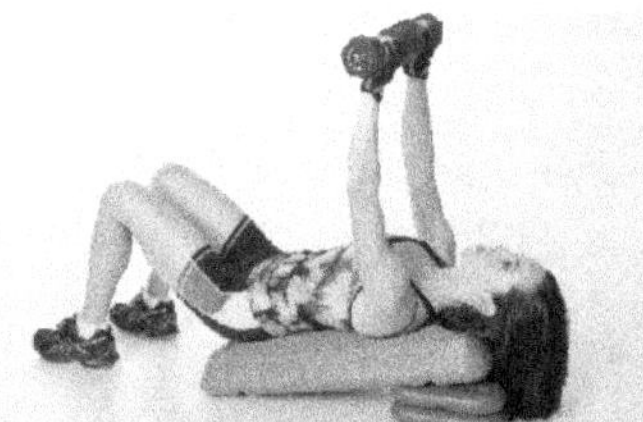 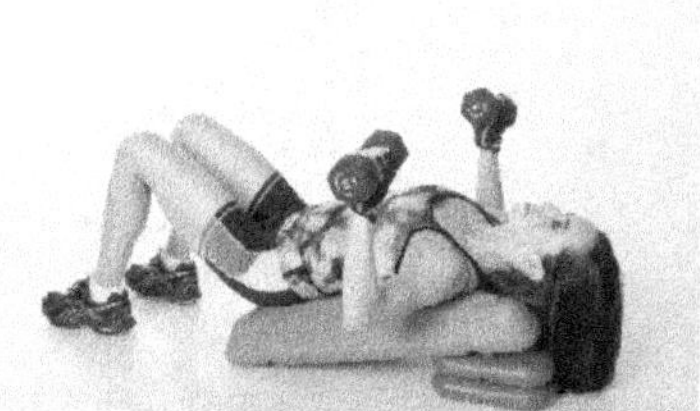

Dumbbell Chest Flys

Lie on a bench with two dumbbells held above your head, at arm's length, facing and touching each other. For the traditional position, the bench is flat on the floor. (This image shows the correct positioning, but the bench has been adjusted for the incline position. You can do the exact same thing with the bench flat.) Inhale as you lower the dumbbells out to each side of your chest, keeping your elbow slightly bent the entire time. Do not lower the weights past your shoulders. Keep your chest high and keep the natural curve in your back.

Exhale as you return to the starting point, again, keeping your elbows slightly bent.

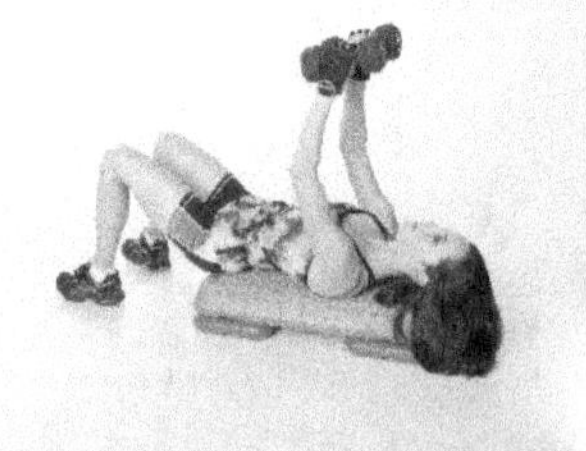 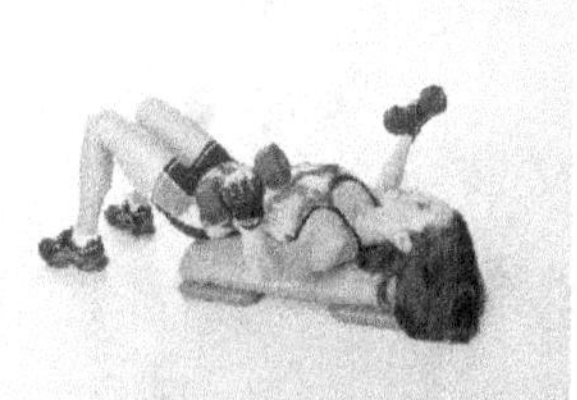

Incline Chest Flys

This move is very similar to the Dumbbell Chest Flys mentioned earlier, but this one is at a slight incline, which helps to work the muscles differently. You always want to vary the stimulus on the muscles you're working and change them up frequently. In this case, the incline puts the focus on the upper part of your chest.

To create an incline, you can do this on an incline bench at the gym, or remove one of the risers from your step bench (as shown here) and put it on the other end, raising the bench slightly. Lie on a bench with two dumbbells held above your head, at arm's length, facing and touching each other. Inhale as you lower the dumbbells out to each side of your chest, keeping your elbow slightly bent the entire time. Do not lower the weights past your shoulders. Keep your chest high and keep the natural curve in your back. Exhale as you return to the starting point, again keeping your elbows slightly bent.

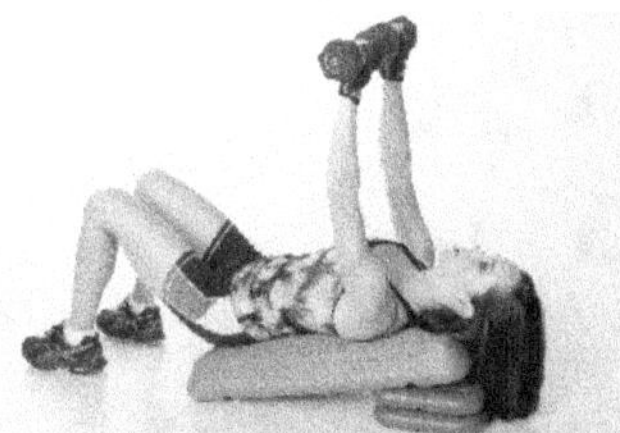 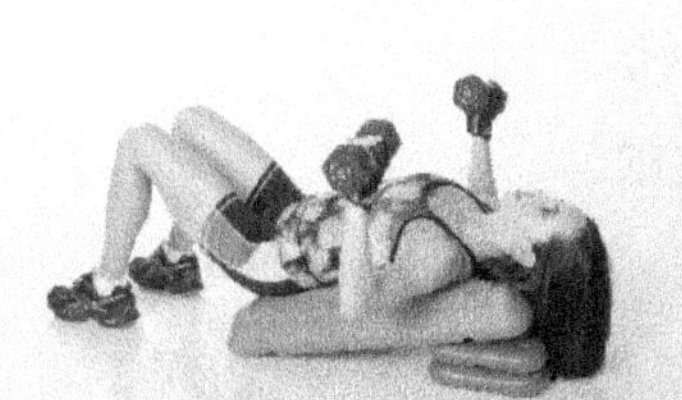

Standing Pec Dec

Stand shoulder-width apart with your knees slightly bent. Hold two dumbbells facing outward with your arms bent in 90-degree angles out to the sides. Inhale as you pull your arms in leading with the elbows. Exhale as you bring them back to the starting position.

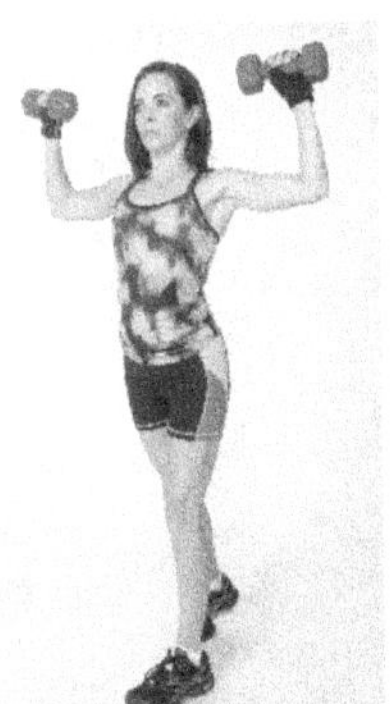 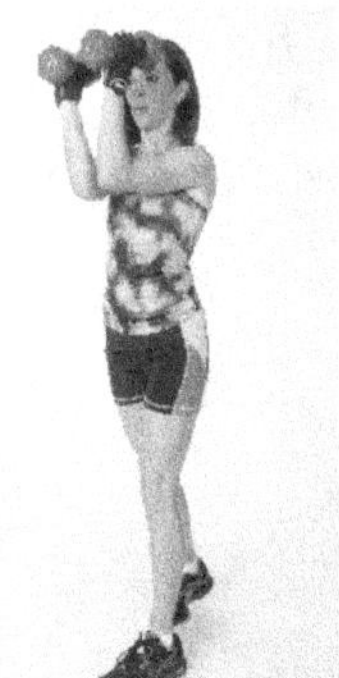 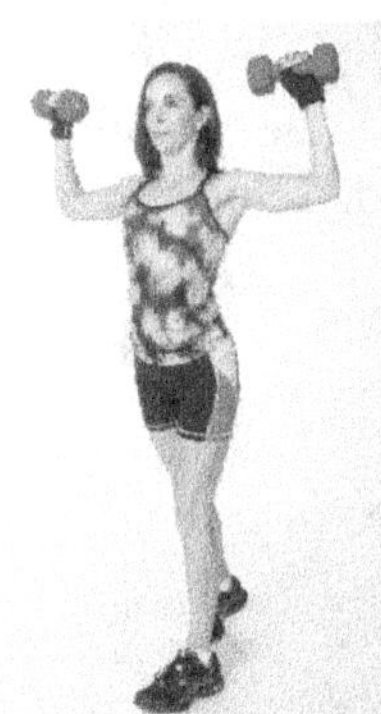

Pushups

You can do pushups on your knees or toes, but make sure you maintain a wide, stable open-palm grip and force your weight slightly forward so you work the chest and shoulders properly.

Starting at the top, inhale as you come down until your chest is right above the floor. Exhale as you push up. To do this exercise on your knees, simply place your knees side by side on the floor and keep your back straight.

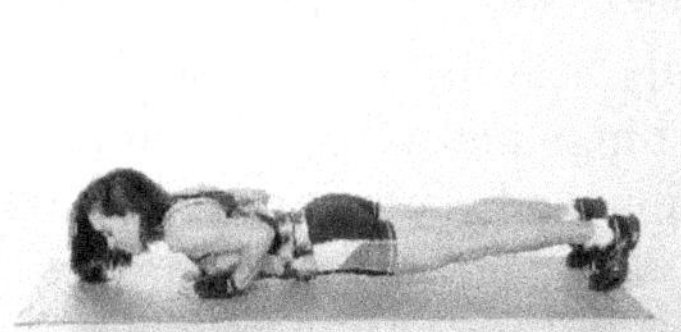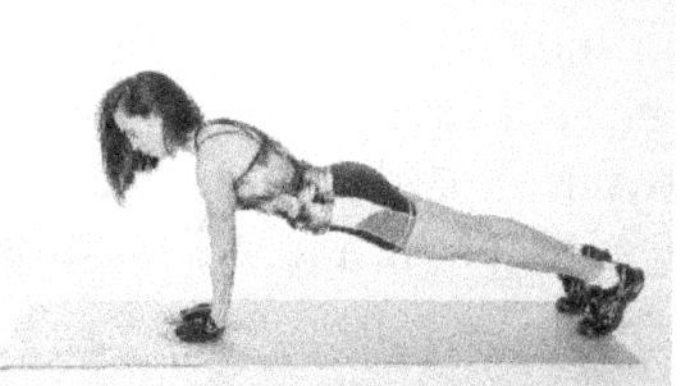

SHOULDERS

Dumbbell Lateral Raises

Standing in set position (knees slightly bent and feet about shoulder-width apart), hold two dumbbells in front of your thighs and facing one another.

Tipping slightly forward at the waist so the dumbbells clear your thighs, inhale as you bring the weights up and out to the sides with your arms slightly bent.

At the top position, the dumbbells should be slightly higher than your shoulders, but be careful not to compromise the positioning of your form by raising your shoulders at the top. Inhale as you lift the weights, and exhale as you return them to the starting position.

> **FIT MOM TIP:**
>
> For additional stability, you can also change your standing position to the split stance so that one foot is slightly back as a support.

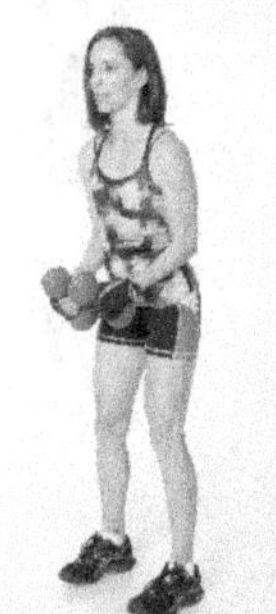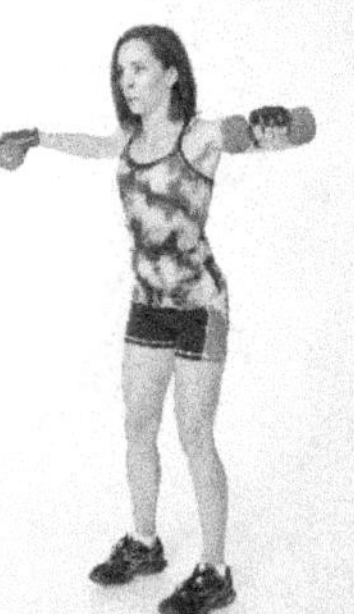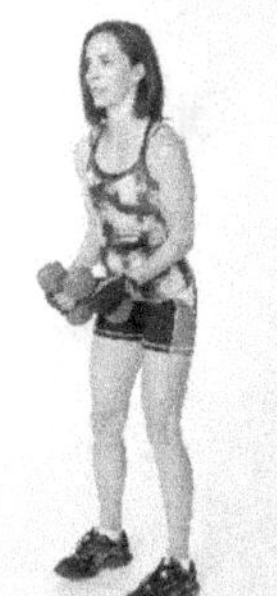

Front Raises

Stand in set position (knees slightly bent and feet about shoulder-width apart). Hold two dumbbells in front of your thighs and with your palms facing your body. Tighten your abdominal muscles and inhale as you bring both dumbbells up with your arms fully extended, stopping at shoulder height.

Exhale as you bring them back to the starting position, keeping the focus on the shoulder muscle on the way down. You can also do alternating front raises (one at a time), as shown here.

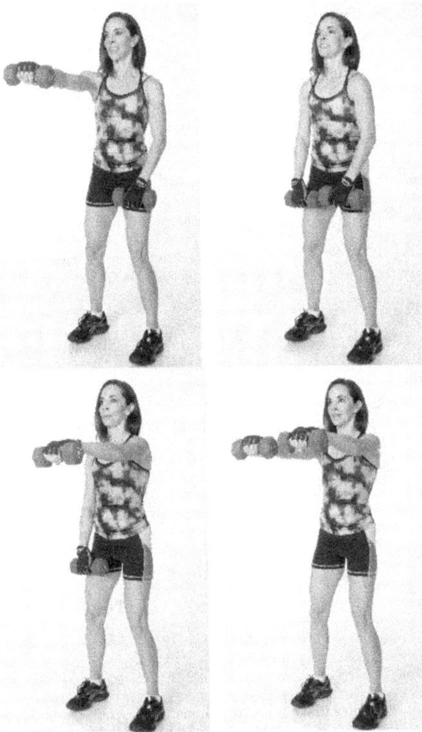

FIT MOM TIP:

My shoulders are typically weaker than other muscle groups, so I have to drop down the weight. For example, if I lift 12 pounds for biceps, I typically have to go as low as 8 pounds for this shoulder exercise. It might take a while to find the right weight for the right muscle group, so just play around with it to find which ones work best for you. Rule of thumb: the last three repetitions of any exercise should be difficult but not impossible. If you can do three sets easily, then it's time to move up in weights!

Seated Shoulder Press

Sit on a workout bench or chair with your feet flat on the ground. Hold two dumbbells out to the sides in 90-degree angles, palms facing out. Exhale as you push the weights up and over your head until they barely touch at the top. Inhale as you bring them back to the starting position.

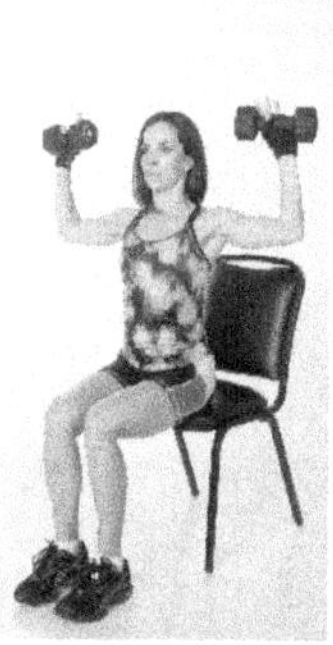 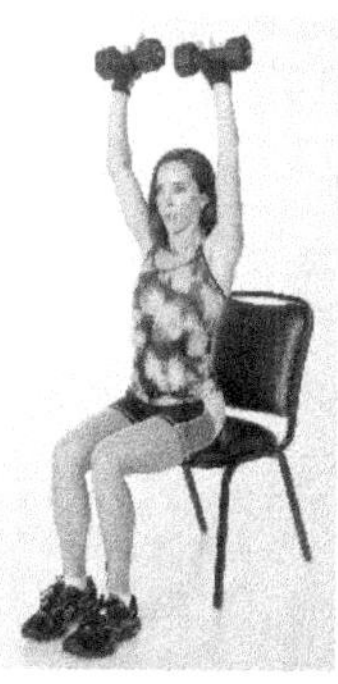 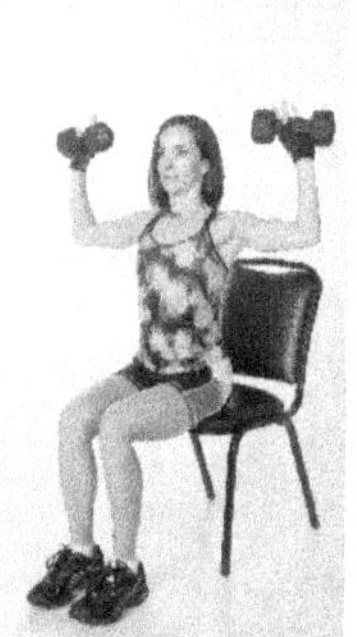

Wide Squat with Front Raises

Stand with your feet out past your shoulders and toes pointed slightly outward. Hold two dumbbells and then exhale as you squat straight down until your thighs are parallel to the floor. As you squat down, raise the dumbbells forward until they are shoulder level. Inhale as you come back to the original position. Resist swinging the weights or letting them drop back into place.

The work is in feeling the resistance as you raise your arms up and down.

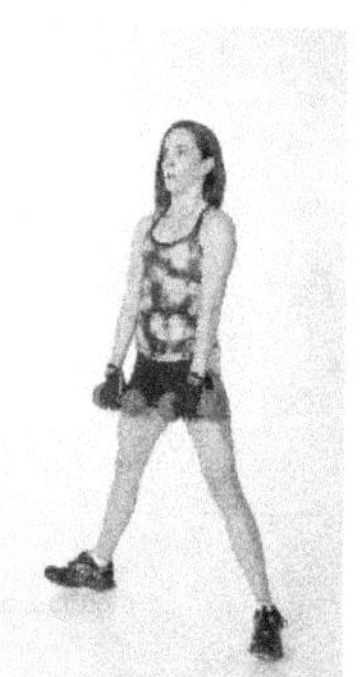 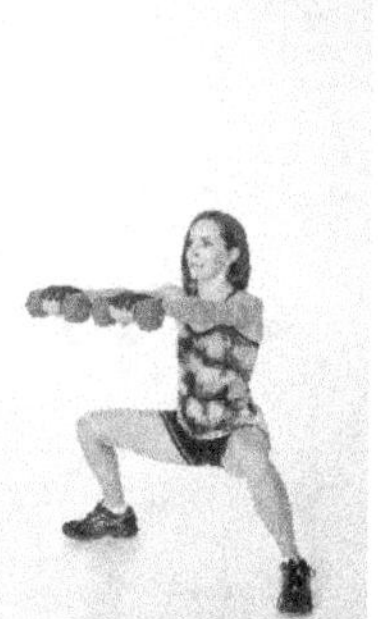 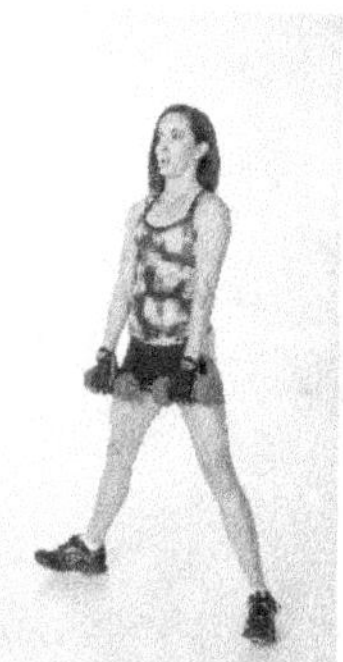

FIT MOM TIP:

This is a compound move that works the shoulders, legs and glutes at the same time, which makes it a great timesaver exercise! But it also means it will bring your heart rate up higher than if you did a traditional set of standing front raises. The extra cardio will help you burn more calories within a shorter period of time.

Standing Shoulder Rotators

Stand with your feet about shoulder-width apart. Hold two medium to light dumbbells and set your position with your arms out to the sides and in 90-degree angles.

Inhale as you rotate your elbows forward, keeping everything else completely still. Keep your arms in 90-degree angles and stop the move when your palms are facing the floor.

Exhale as you rotate them back up to the starting position.

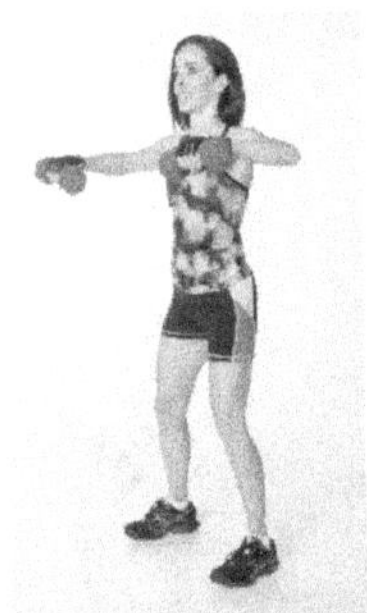
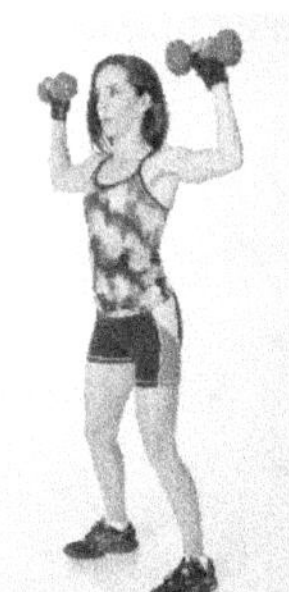
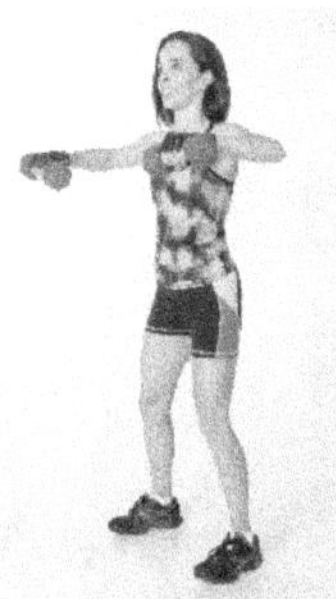

FIT MOM TIP:

Since as I've said, shoulders tend to be one of my weaker muscle groups, I do this exercise using 8 or 5 pound dumbbells. You can start with 5's and work your way up. Be careful to keep the top shoulder muscles completely neutral and don't let them sneak up to your ears!

Standing Push-Press

This is a compound movement because you're working two major muscle groups simultaneously – the shoulders and legs. Involving the legs means you can go a little heavier with the weighted dumbbells because you're going to use your legs to help you push up.

Stand with your feet shoulder-width apart. Hold two heavy dumbbells close to your body and at shoulder level. Inhale as you squat down. Exhale as you push up, keeping your knees slightly bent and pushing both arms overhead.

Do not lock your elbows. Inhale as you return to the squat position and bring the weights back to shoulder level.

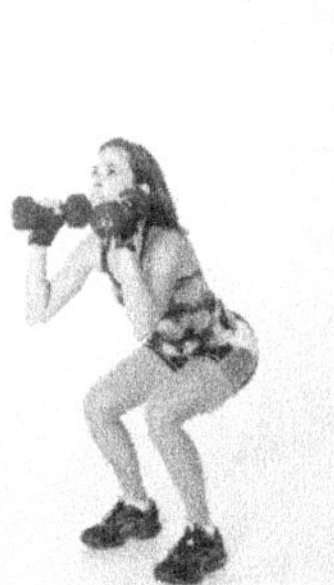
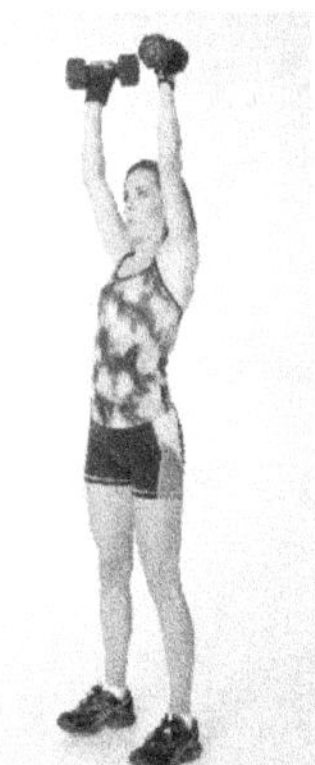

LEGS & GLUTES

Standing Squat

> **FIT MOM TIP:**
>
> To vary the exercise and clear the weights from bumping your thighs and hips, you can put the dumbbells on top of your shoulders as shown here. This forces the weight to the center, making it easier to balance. I prefer this position, as it makes me feel more stable and less likely to injure myself because I'm more secure.

Stand shoulder-width apart with your feet facing forward. Hold two dumbbells at your sides with your palms facing in.

Inhale as you lower your body, pushing your bottom back like you're sitting in a chair. Try to get your thighs parallel to the floor. Keep your head and chest up for the entire motion. Exhale as you push up, but be careful not to lock the knees. Keep your knees slightly bent the entire time and force your weight into your heels as you lower and rise up again.

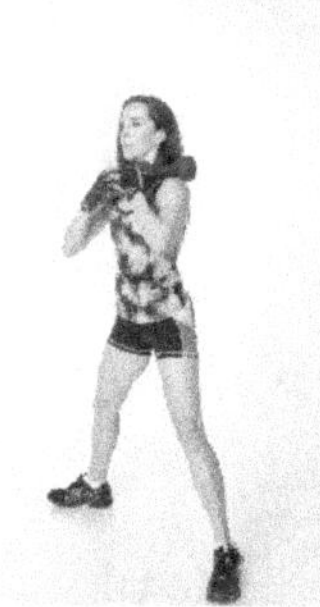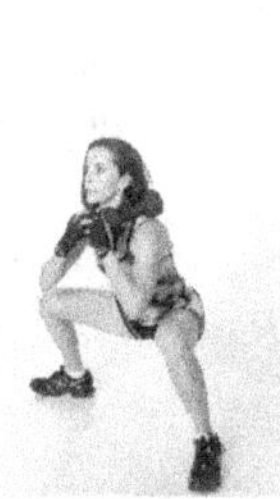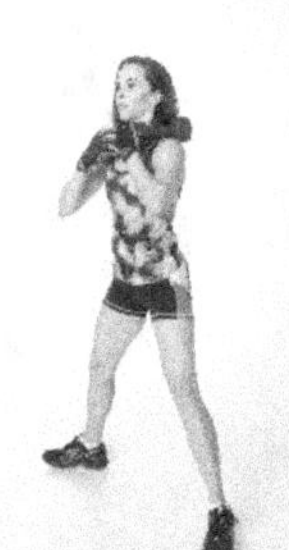

Wide Squat

This move is similar to the Standing Squat, but you stand with your feet further apart than shoulder-width and feet turned slightly out. It's your choice if you want to hold two dumbbells at your sides or place them on top of your shoulders (as shown here), but I've personally found the latter to be easier because I don't bang my thighs on the descent.

Inhale and push your bottom back, keeping your head and chest up. Go as far as you can until your thighs are parallel to the floor. Exhale as you push up, forcing all the weight into your heels and keeping your knees slightly bent the entire time.

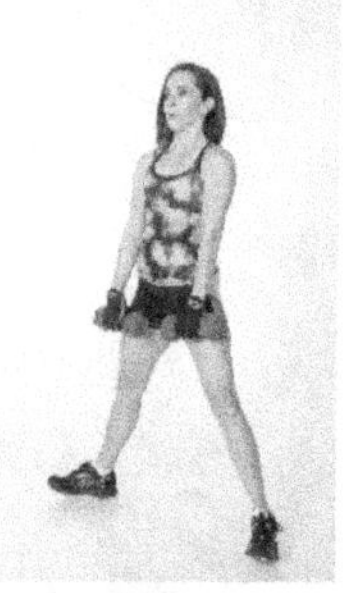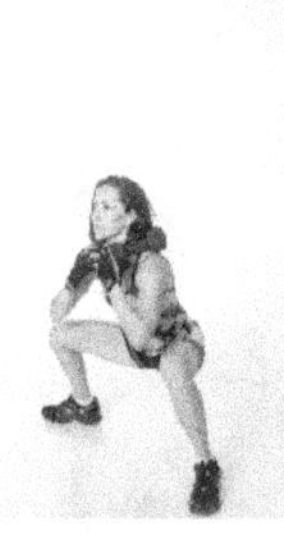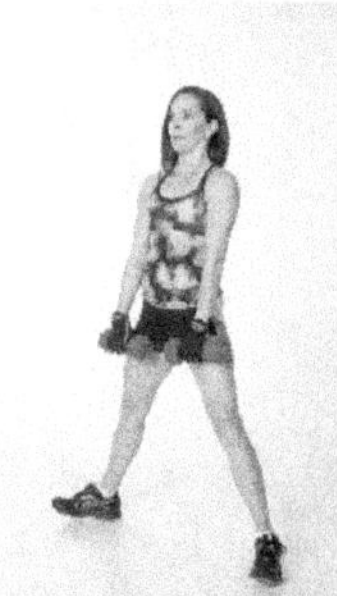

Lunges on Bench

There are many varieties of the traditional lunge. This one, where one foot is elevated on the bench, is more intense and puts more stress on the quadriceps of the forward lunging leg. In general, the longer your lunge step, the more the hamstrings will be used, and the shorter the step, the more focus on the quadriceps. But the most important thing to remember with this exercise is how to place the forward foot relative to your knee and to not lunge where your knee passes your toes.

Stand with two dumbbells either down at your sides or placed on your shoulders. Place one foot on your bench and step back with the other foot until you feel stable.

FIT MOM TIP:

Holding the dumbbells on your shoulders forces the weight to the center of your body and helps you to stabilize.

Inhale as you lower your front leg until your thigh is parallel to the floor.

Exhale as you return to the starting position.

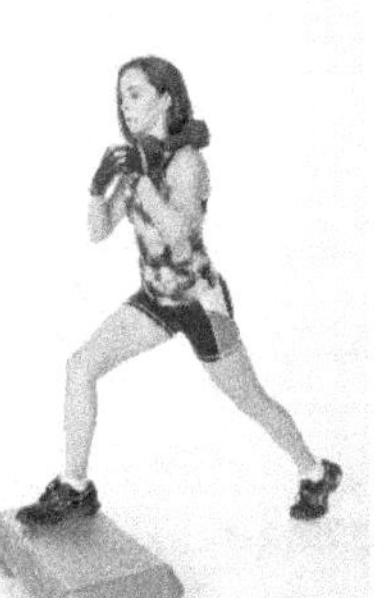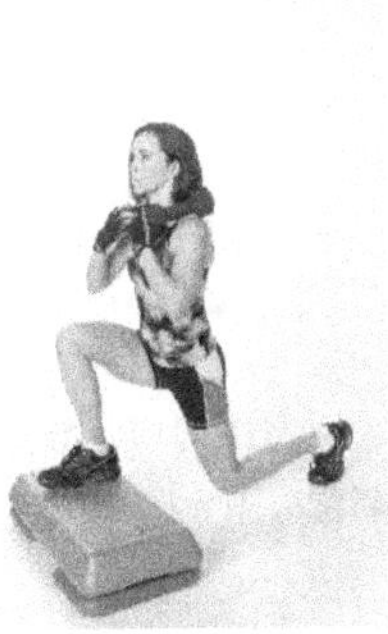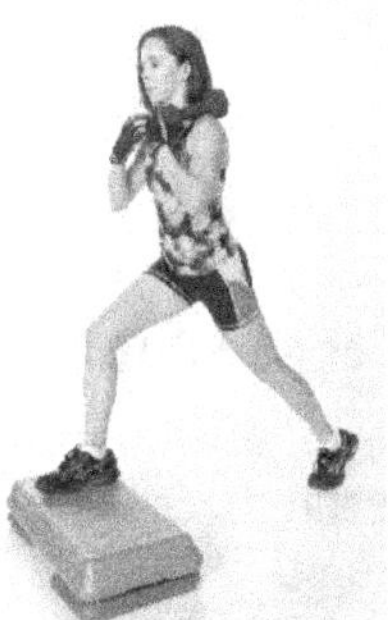

Walking Lunges

Stand with two heavy dumbbells either down at your sides or placed on your shoulders. Step forward into a lunge. You want your front leg to be at a 90-degree angle and your forward thigh to be parallel to the floor. Step together, pause, and repeat, alternating your legs. Inhale as you step forward, and exhale as you come up bringing your back leg to the starting position.

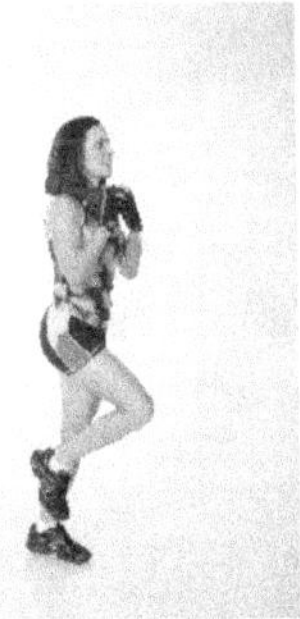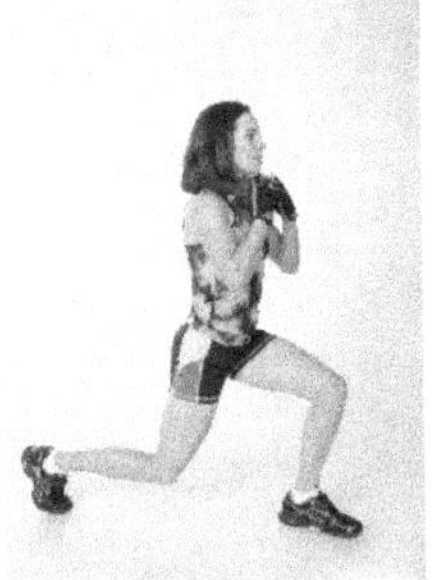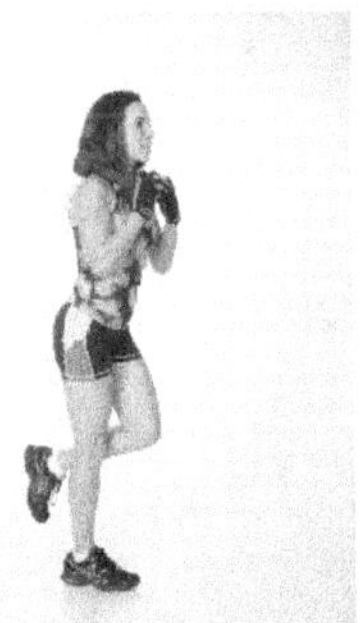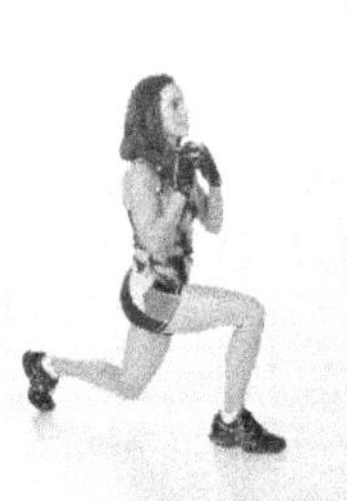

Calf Raises

Stand on top of a workout bench with your heels hanging off the edge. Using just the balls of your feet, push up with your toes. Lower your heels to the lowest point possible for a comfortable stretch. Pause briefly before returning to the top. Pause and repeat. To vary the stress on the calf muscles, you can modify this exercise by doing straight calf raises, then turn your toes toward each other for a set, then turn your heels to each other for a different set.

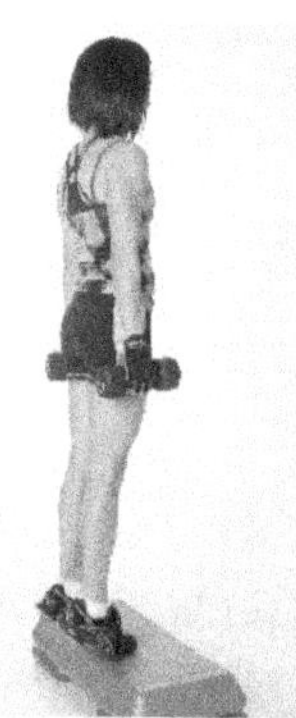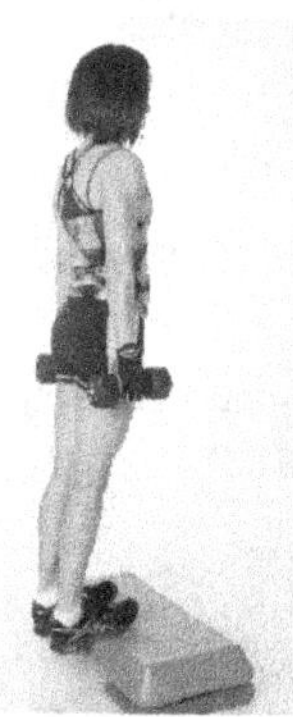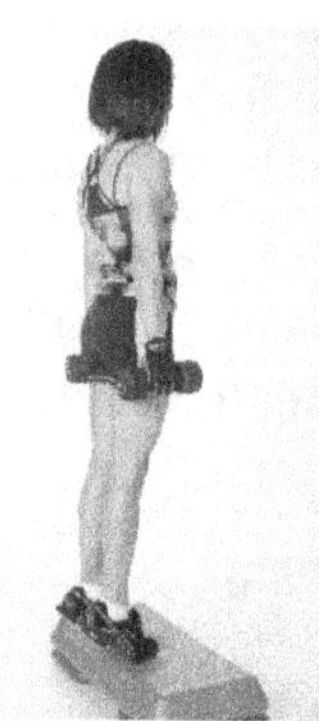

Single Legged Squat

Use the back of a chair for stability for this exercise, but make sure to use the chair only as a stabilizer – don't cheat by letting the chair take your weight rather than your standing leg!

Hold a heavy dumbbell on the same side as your squat leg. Inhale as you squat, being careful to not overextend your knee past your toes. Exhale as you come up, and watch that you keep your knees slightly bent the entire time. Complete a full set and switch legs.

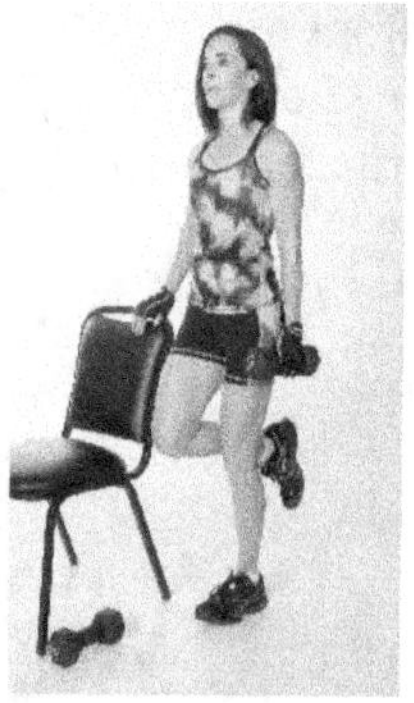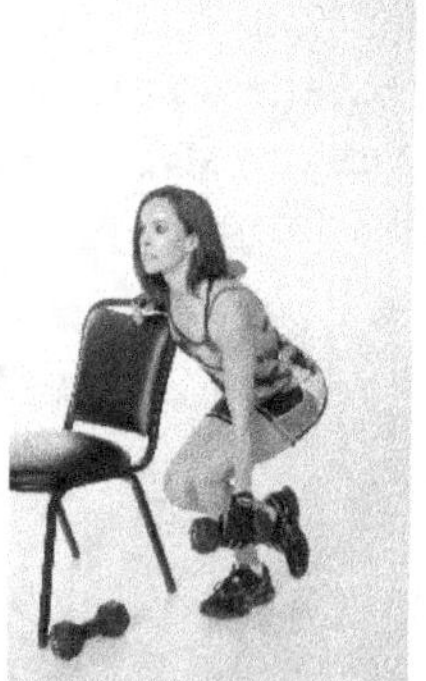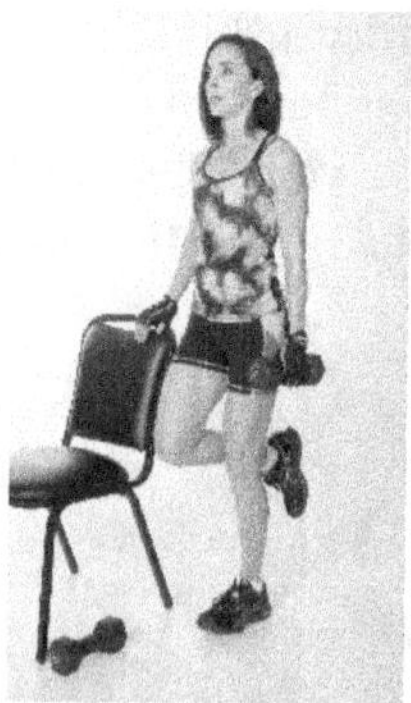

Donkey Kicks

Start on all fours on a soft mat. Place a heavy dumbbell in the crook of one knee and squeeze it into place with your leg. Keep your back straight and exhale as you lift leg and dumbbell into the air. Hold, and inhale as you bring the dumbbell back down. Finish one complete set on one leg and then switch to the other leg.

Warning: The first time I did three sets of 20 of these on each leg, I could barely walk the next day! These are great for strengthening and toning your glutes and hamstrings.

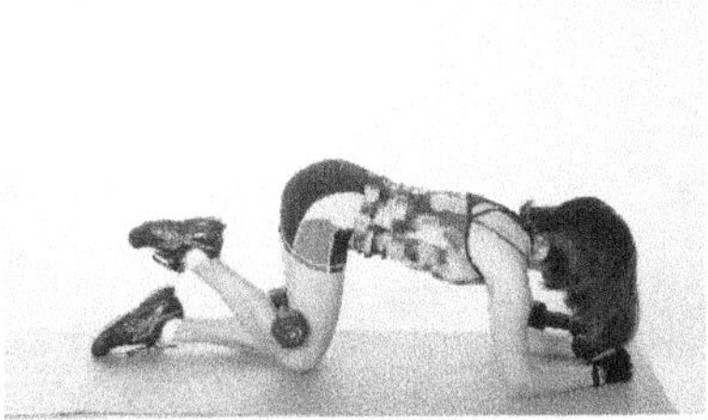 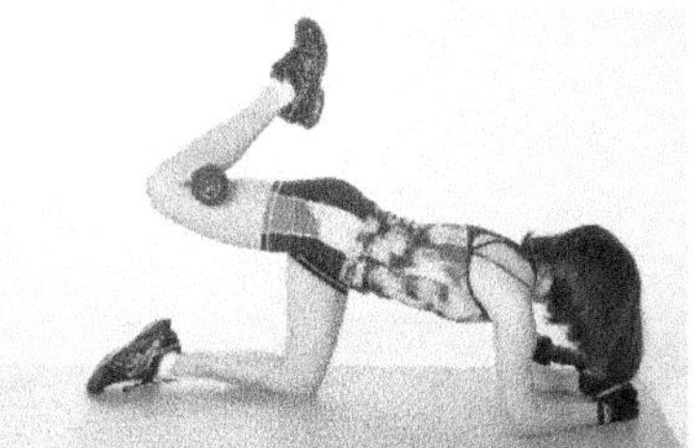

Jump Squats

Stand in a mid-stance squat position, with your feet about shoulder-width apart. Prepare to jump as you inhale and bring your arms down and back. Then, pushing through your heels, jump up, reaching as high as you can toward the ceiling. Land on the center of your foot and back into the squat, as this protects your knees from impact.

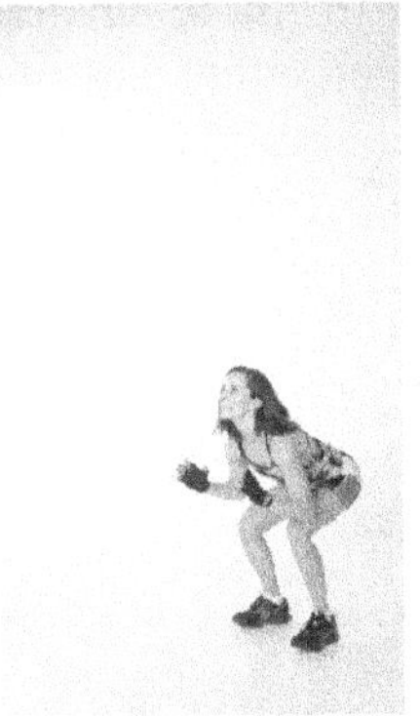 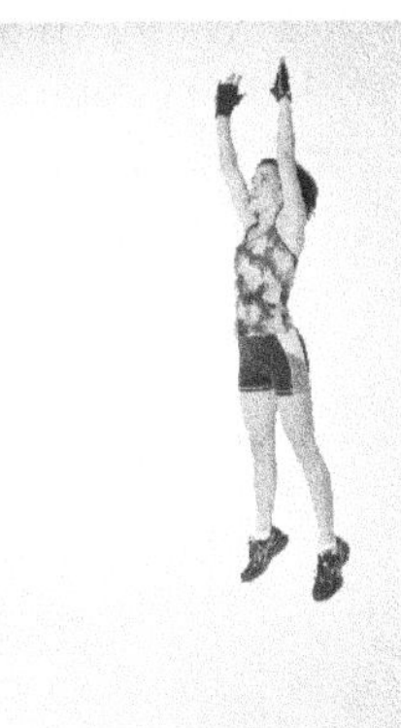 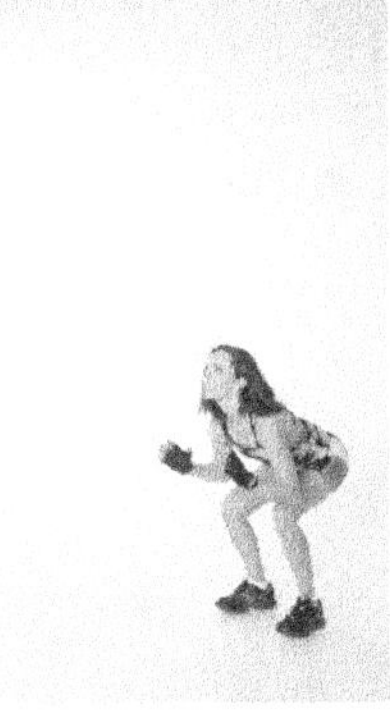

Side-to-Side Plyos

The benefit of working in plyometric exercises in between resistance workouts is to increase your heart rate and burn more calories. Plyometrics, also known as "jump training" or "plyos," are exercises that exert maximum force on the muscle in as short a time as possible, with the goal of increasing both power and speed. The more you add these into your workouts, the quicker you'll recover and drop more leftover baby weight!

Stand with one foot on the floor and the other up on a step bench. Jump up to the top of the bench as you switch feet and come down into a side squat on the other side. Switch and repeat.

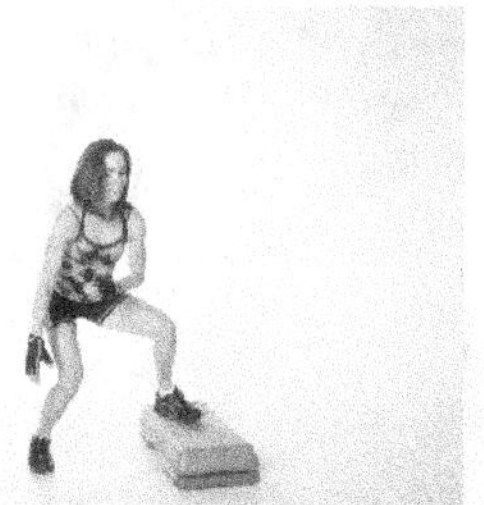 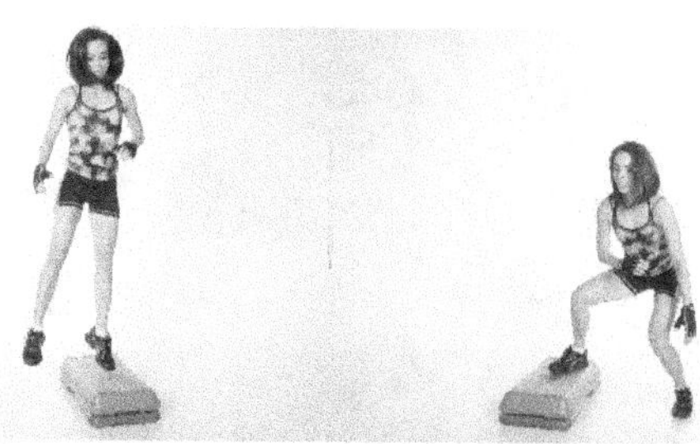

You can do plyos in timed sets of 30 to 45 seconds.

Bench Plyos

Stand with both feet on top of the bench. Using your arms for leverage, jump up and land flat-footed on the ground in a wide squat, one leg on either side of the bench. Pause, then jump back up onto the bench and repeat. Exhale at the greatest point of exertion as you explode off the bench and up into the air. Inhale at the bottom as you repeat the exercise.

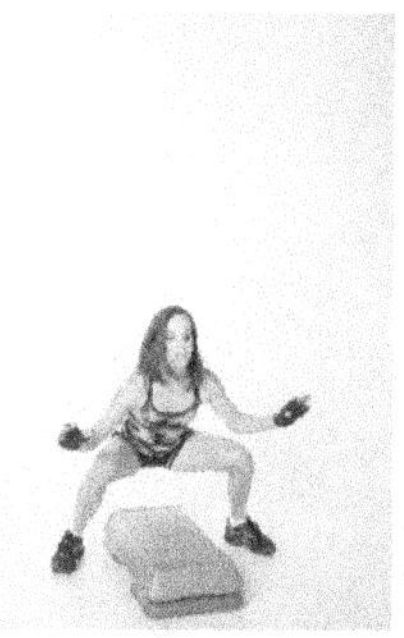 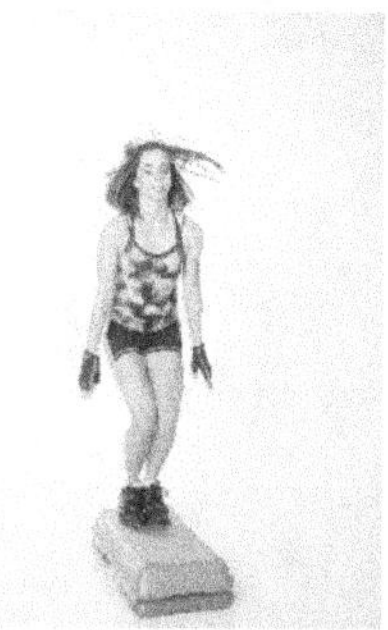 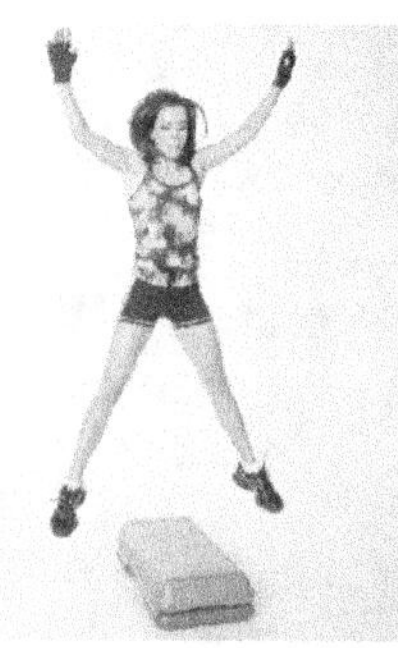 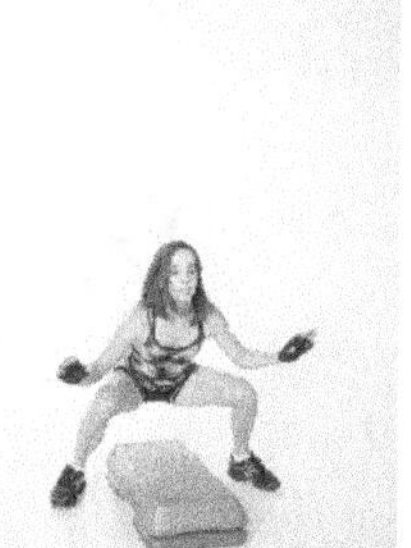

Tuck-Jump Burpees

The burpee is a full body exercise used in strength training and as an aerobic exercise. It is performed in four steps with several variations available. This one contains a tuck jump at the end for an extra caloric burn. These will skyrocket your heart rate, so tread carefully.

1. Start in a squat position with your hands on the floor.
2. Kick your feet out into a pushup position.
3. Quickly, bring both feet back in together.
4. Kick off the floor into a jump and bring your knees into your chest at the top (tuck position).
5. Land flat on your feet with a bend in your knees.

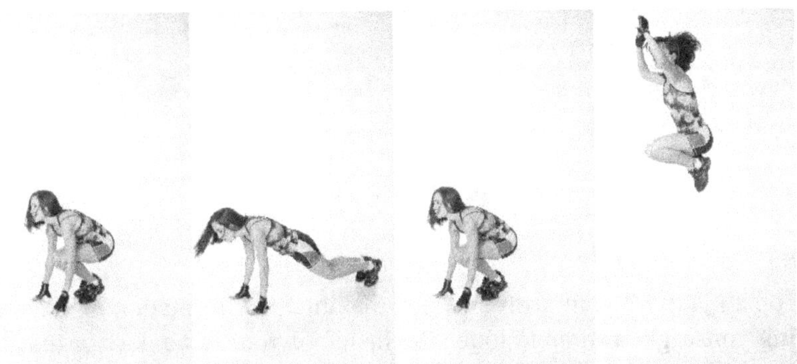

ABS

Crunches

Lie down on a mat with your knees bent and feet planted firmly on the ground. Place your hands gently behind your head, but be careful not to use them to pull your neck forward as you come up. Exhale as you crunch up, pulling in your bellybutton and squeezing your abdominal muscles. Inhale as you return to the starting position, but keep your head and neck up off the floor.

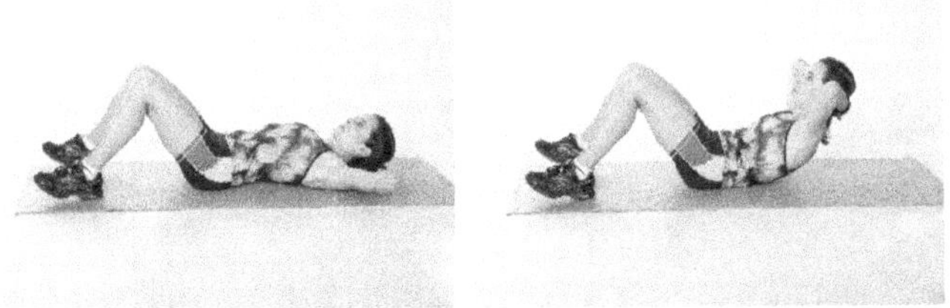

Sit-ups with Weight

FIT MOM TIP:

Be careful not to use the momentum of the weight to pull you forward and backward or you're not really getting the benefit of the exercise. A dumbbell or plate that weighs between 8 and 12 pounds is good for this exercise.

As with the crunch, you start by lying on a mat with your knees bent and feet planted firmly on the ground. Hold a dumbbell or weighted barbell plate over your head in both hands.

Exhale as you squeeze up, pulling in your bellybutton and lifting the dumbbell toward the ceiling as you rise to a sitting position. Inhale as you return to position.

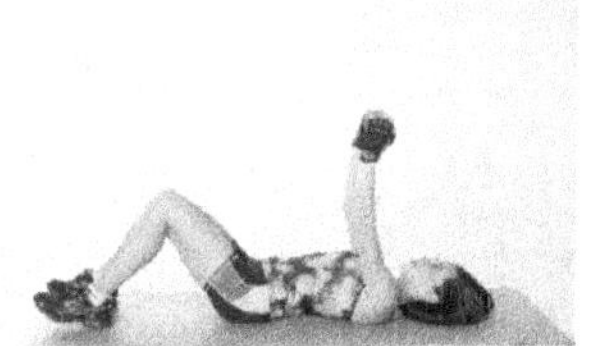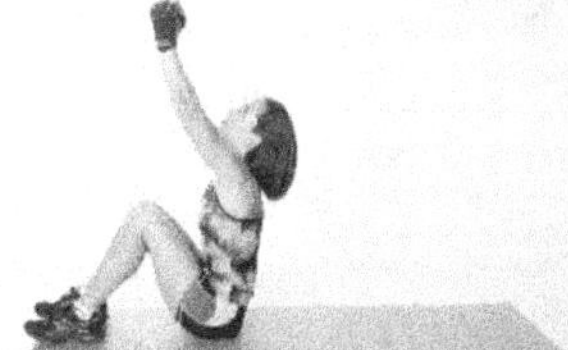

Starfishes

Lie down on a mat with your arms and legs making an X formation on the mat. Exhale as you bring your right arm up to touch the inside of your left ankle (or toes if you can reach that far). Squeeze your abdominal muscles as you come up – it feels like you're pulling your bellybutton all the way in. Inhale as you come back down. Alternate sides and this time exhale as you bring your left arm up to the inside of your right ankle.

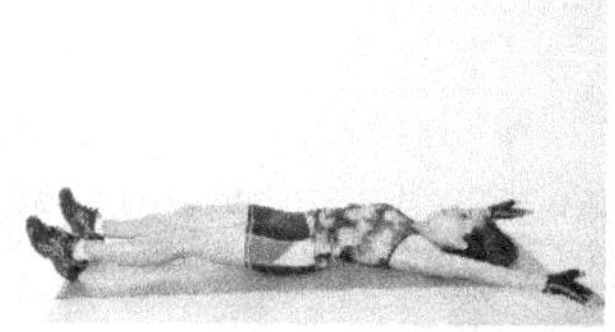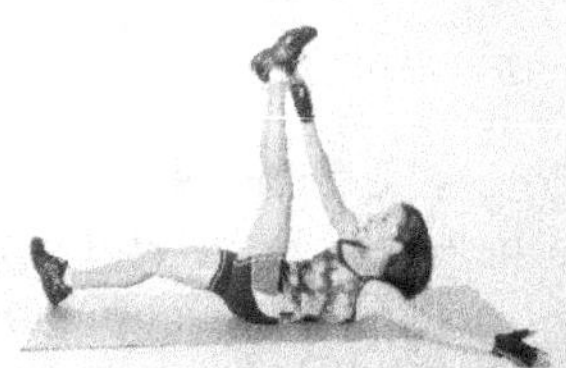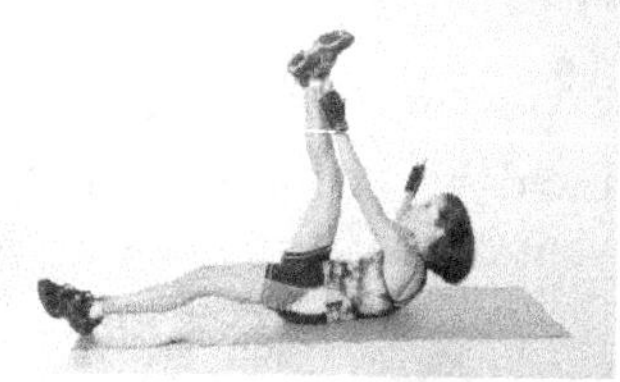

Crisscrosses

This works best as a timed exercise. The longer the time for the exercise, the more difficult it becomes. For example, first set a timer for 30 seconds and perform three sets, resting for 15 seconds in between. When you're strong enough, set the timer for 45 seconds or 60 seconds, etc. Perform three sets of your predetermined timed amount.

Exhale as you crunch, bringing in your bellybutton. Lift both legs and crisscross them in the air. Make sure to breathe!

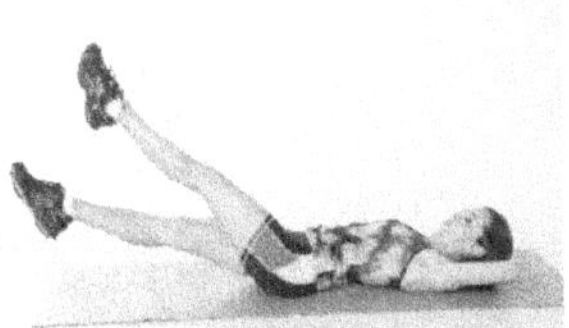 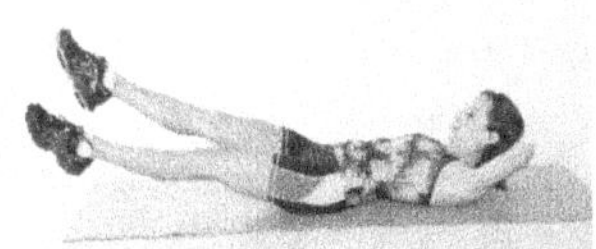

Bicycles

Lie down on a mat with your hands placed gently behind your head and legs outstretched in front of you. Bring your right elbow up to your left knee, exhaling as you reach the top of the exercise. Inhale as you switch to the other side.

Continue alternating bicycles, either for a timed exercise or in three sets of 20.

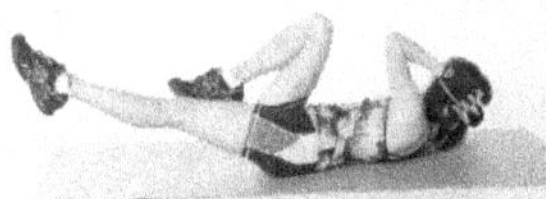 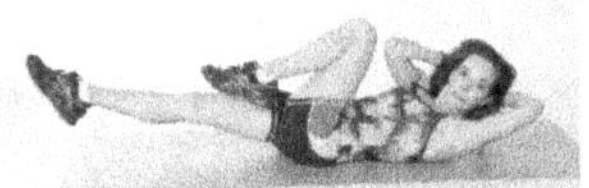

Planks

There are several versions to this exercise – you can come all the way up onto your hands or do them on your forearms, as shown. To make them even more difficult, elevate your toes on a step bench while you maintain the plank formation on your forearms. The object is to keep your body completely straight, like a board. Hold in 30-second or 60-second intervals.

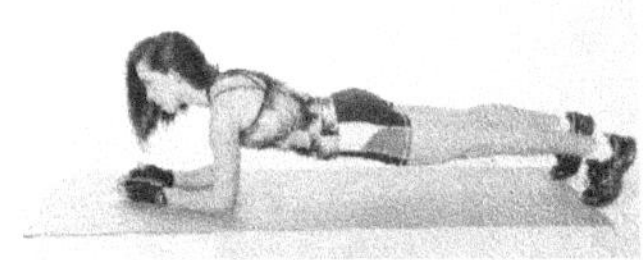

Reverse Crunches

Lie flat on a mat placed on the floor. Put your hands down at your sides, either on the mat or behind your buttocks with your palms facing down. Inhale as you bring your legs up while squeezing your abdominal muscles and pulling in your bellybutton. Exhale as you slowly return to the starting position.

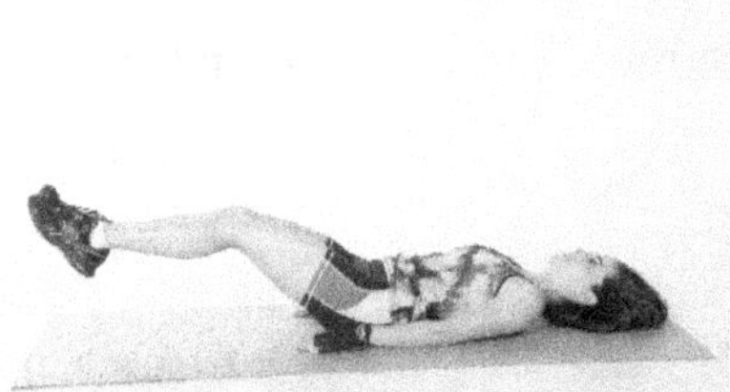 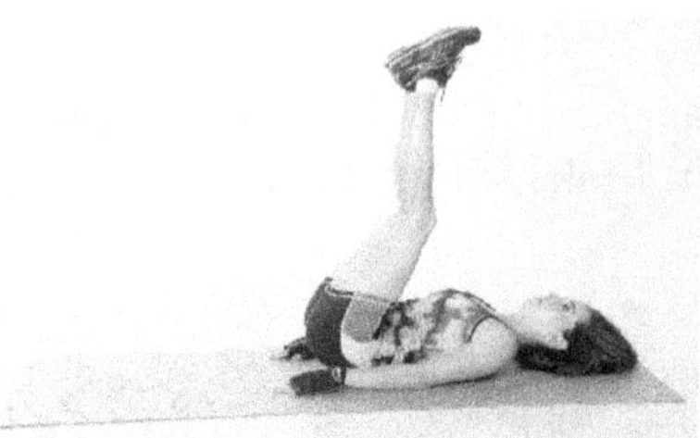

Plank Twists

Lie on one side with your elbow on the floor and shoulders above your elbow. Lift your body weight up using your elbow and shoulder to manage most of the weight. You can do this on your knees or up on your toes. Bring your free arm under your body, rotating inward. Pause, inhale as you bring the arm up and lift it toward the ceiling. Exhale as you pull it back in for the twist. Do three sets of 12 on each side.

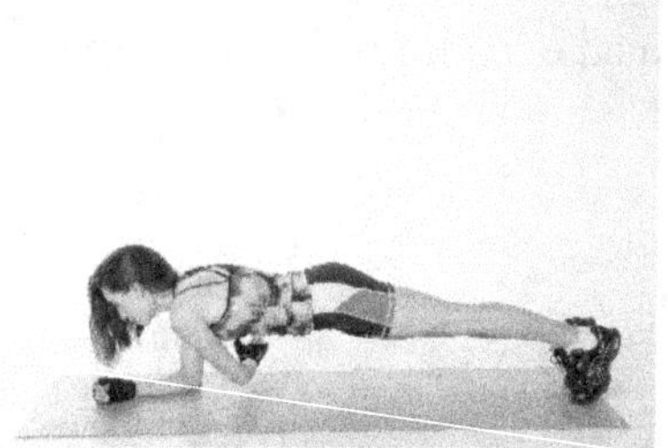 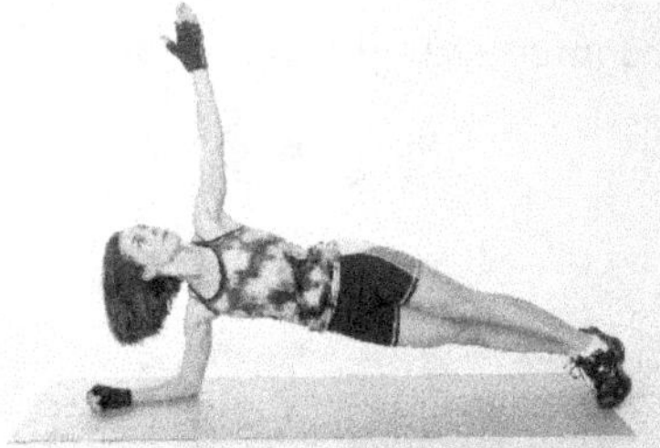

Oblique Crunches

Lie on a mat with your knees turned to the side. Place your hands gently behind your head. Exhale as you lift your neck and shoulders up off the floor. Inhale as you release, but keep your head and neck up off the floor while performing the exercise.

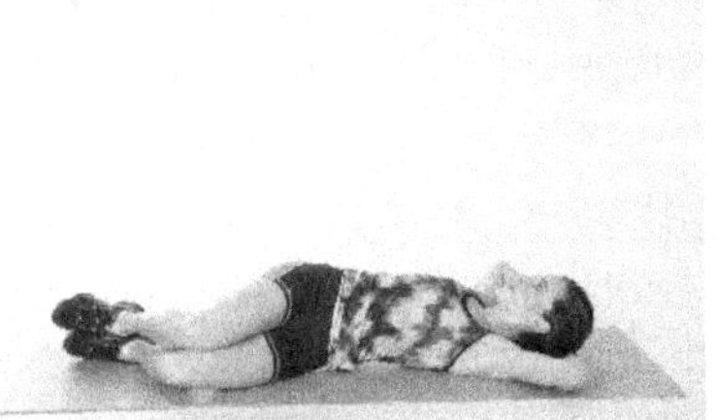
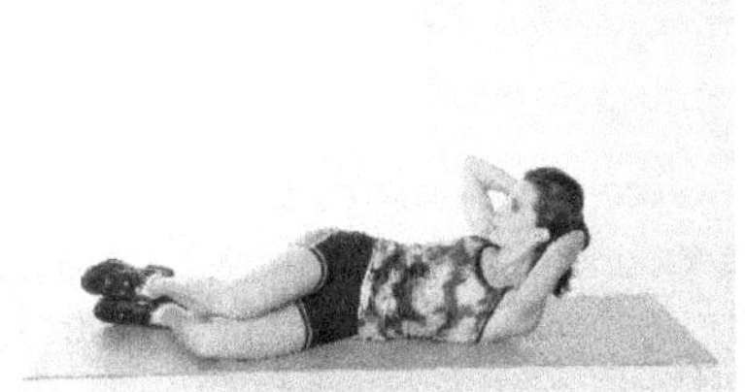

Russian Twists

On a mat on the floor, position your body so your upper body creates a V shape relative to your thighs. Hold a heavy plate or dumbbell in front of your chest with both hands. Twist your torso to one side as you exhale and bring the weight down, almost to the floor. Hold the contraction. Inhale in the neutral position or when the weight is centered to your body. Switch to the other side and exhale.

FIT MOM TIP:

Holding a weighted dumbbell or plate is an advanced move. If you're not quite ready for that yet, simply perform the exercise without any weight at all.

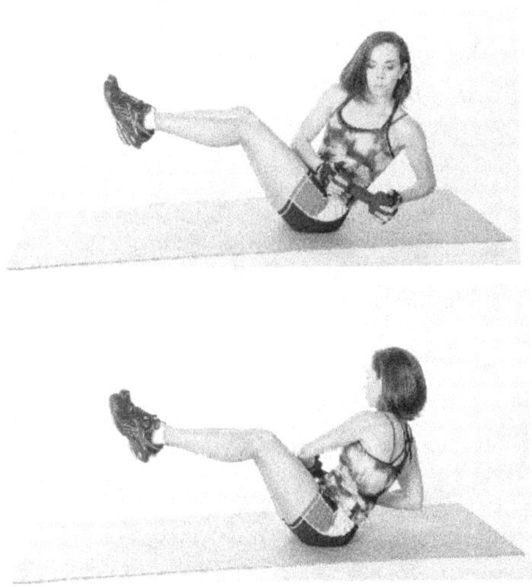

Advanced Twelve-Week Workout

Remember to rest about one minute in between sets, as long as it takes for your breathing to return to normal. The break in between exercises should be as long as it takes you to set up the next machine or sets of weights for that body part, generally three to five minutes. Do one set of each exercise for warm-up, then do each exercise three times, or for three sets, twelve – fifteen reps each. Warm-up should take about five minutes. Stretch the muscle groups you worked at the end of every workout.

You'll notice that some of the exercises listed say "high risk" next to them. A high-risk exercise is one that can be dangerous for someone who is predisposed for having an injury that pertains to the particular muscle group the exercise works. For example, someone with a previous back injury should proceed with caution before doing any of the deadlifts or hyperextensions. High risk exercises are best for those who are familiar with the exercise itself, i.e., an advanced person who has done resistance training in the past and who is comfortable with their form. High risk doesn't mean "stay away," but it simply means "be aware and do it correctly."

If you're not sure about your form, ask a personal trainer friend to watch you for one or two reps and make sure to watch yourself in a bathroom mirror or in front of reflective glass to make sure you're set up properly. I'm a huge advocate of doing exercises in a slow, consistent fashion so you have longevity with your fitness. After all, this isn't just to hit a short-term goal – you also want to be able to do these exercises and maintain your level of fitness for the rest of your life. That's my goal anyway!

If you want more personalized attention with the interactive version of this program with support and motivation, you can sign up for the affordable Super Mom Get Fit Program risk-free at *www.FitMomSecrets.com/Book-Offer*.

Week 1

Day of the Week		Exercises
Monday	Back and Biceps, Abs	Bent-over Dumbbell Row
		One-arm Dumbbell Row
		Barbell Deadlift (*high risk)
		Standing Dumbbell Curl
		Standing Hammer Dumbbell Curl
		3 Sets of Bent Knee Crunches
		3 Sets of In-and-Outs
		3 Sets of Starfishes

Tuesday	Chest, Shoulders and Triceps	Dumbbell Bench Press
		Flat Flys
		20 Push-ups (on toes if you can)
		Standing Dumbbell Press
		Dumbbell Side Laterals
		Standing Barbell Press (*high risk)
		Triceps Extension
		Bench-Dips (*high risk)
		20 Triceps push-ups
Wednesday	Rest	Moms with babies: stroller walk for 45 minutes
		Moms with older kids: Cardio on treadmill or stationary bike for 45 minutes
Thursday	Legs, Abs	Squats (standard and wide)
		Lunges with Dumbbells
		Donkey Kicks
		Standing Calf Raises with Dumbbells
		20 Reverse Crunches x 3
		20 In and Outs x 3 with a dumbbell
		Ab Crunches x 3
Friday	Cardio	Kickboxing class or run sprints outside for 45 minutes
Saturday	Back and Biceps	Wide-grip Lat Pull-downs (*high risk)
		Bent-over Dumbbell Rows
		Barbell Deadlifts (*high risk)
		Extended Dumbbell Curls
		Concentration Dumbbell Curls
		Standing Hammer Curls
Sunday	Rest	Cardio on treadmill for 45 minutes

Week 2

Day of the Week		Exercises
Monday	Chest, Shoulders and Triceps	Barbell Bench Press
		Incline Bench Press with Dumbbells
		Pec Dec (*high risk)
		Standing Front Raises
		Bent-over Side Laterals
		Sitting Shoulder Press with Dumbbells
		Triceps Extension (Heavy weight)
		Overhead Dumbbell (Single Arm)
		Triceps kick-backs
Tuesday	Legs, Abs	Warm up legs by marching in place and doing side-to-side steps for 5 minutes or by jogging outside for 10 minutes
		Plié squats
		Single legged squats
		Walking lunges with dumbbells
		Leg Presses
		Side plank twists x 3
		Reverse crunches with an exercise ball x 3
		Hold plank on toes for 1 minute, rest 1 minute x 3
Wednesday	Rest	Moms with babies: stroller walk for 45 minutes
		Moms with older kids: Cardio on treadmill or stationary bike for 45 minutes

Thursday	Back and Biceps	Deadlifts with Triple Rows (*high risk)
		Reverse grip Deadlift Rows (*high risk)
		Single Arm rows
		Bent-over Dumbbell Rows
		21s x 3
		Hammer Curls
		Switch to plate lifts and twist at the top
		Regular bicep curls to failure for last set
Friday	Cardio	25 Minutes elliptical trainer; 25 Minutes running on treadmill
Saturday	Chest, Shoulders and Triceps	5 Minute Warm-up Marching with Arms
		Dumbbell Bench Press
		Dumbbell Flys on Bench
		Incline Dumbbell Press
		Standing Shoulder Press
		Standing Barbell Press (*high risk)
		Standing Side Laterals
		20 Tricep Push-ups x 3
		Lying Barbell Extension (narrow grip) (*high risk)
		Chair or Bench Dips
Sunday	Rest	(Optional) Moms with babies: stroller walk for 45 minutes
		Moms with older kids: Cardio on treadmill or stationary bike for 45 minutes

Week 3

Day of the Week		Exercises
Monday	Legs, Abs (Big muscle groups)	Standing Squats with Barbell
		Standing Squats with Ball on the Wall (go lower to 90 degrees)
		Reverse Lunges on Bench with Dumbbells (use 12s or 15s or more)
		One Set of Stationary Lunges to Failure (no added weight)
		Jump Squats x 3
		Oblique Crunches x 3
		Slow Bicycles x 3
		Slow Straight-Legged Sit-ups x 3
Tuesday	Back and Biceps	Wide-grip Lat Pulldowns (*high risk)
		Seated Cable or Dumbbell Rows
		Wide-grip Deadlift Rows (*high risk)
		Alternate Bicep Curls with Dumbbells
		Alternate Hammer Curls
		Band Bicep Curls
Wednesday	Rest	Moms with babies: stroller walk for 45 minutes
		Moms with older kids: Cardio on treadmill or stationary bike for 45 minutes
Thursday	Chest, Shoulders and Triceps	Cardio warm-up for 5 Minutes
		20 Wide-grip Push-ups
		Barbell Chest Presses
		Incline Dumbbell Presses
		Standing Shoulder Presses
		Standing Lateral Raises
		Plié Squats with Front Raises
		Triceps Kick-backs
		Triceps Extension
		Bench Dips to Failure x 1 (modify)

Friday	Cardio	Turbo kickboxing or interval training with plyos
Saturday	Legs, Abs (Smaller muscle groups)	Stationary Lunges with Dumbbells
		Plié Squats
		Lateral Lunges with Heavy Dumbbell
		Seated Ball Squeezes
		Band Side-to-Side Walks
		3 Sets of Bent Knee Crunches
		3 Sets of In-and-Outs
		3 Sets of Starfishes
Sunday	Rest	Moms with babies: stroller walk for 45 minutes
		Moms with older kids: Cardio on treadmill or stationary bike for 45 minutes

Week 4

Day of the Week		Exercises
Monday	Legs, Abs (Big muscle groups)	Bent-over Dumbbell Row
		One-arm Dumbbell Row
		Barbell Deadlifts (*high risk)
		Standing Dumbbell Curl
		Standing Hammer Dumbbell Curl
		Bent-Knee Crunches x 3
		Tabata Drill x 3 – scissors, swimmers, starfishes
Tuesday	Chest, Shoulders and Triceps	Dumbbell Bench Press
		Flat Flys
		Pec Dec / Rotators
		Standing Dumbbell Press
		Dumbbell Side Laterals (arms bent)
		Dumbbell Side Laterals (arms extended)
		20 Triceps Push-ups x 3
		Lying Barbell Extension (narrow grip)
		Overhead Dumbbell Extension
Wednesday	Rest	Moms with babies: stroller walk for 45 minutes
		Moms with older kids: Cardio on treadmill or stationary bike for 45 minutes
Thursday	Legs, Abs	Squats
		Stationary Lunges w/ Dumbbells
		Donkey Kicks
		Standing Calf Raises with Dumbbells (3 angles)
		20 Reverse Crunches x 3
		20 In and Outs x 3 with a dumbbell
		Ab crunches x 3
Friday	Cardio	Turbo kickboxing class or interval sprints on the treadmill

Saturday	Back and Biceps	Overhead Lat Pull-downs (*high risk)
		Bent-over Dumbbell Rows
		Barbell Deadlifts (*high risk)
		Extended Dumbbell Curls
		Concentration Dumbbell Curls
		Standing Hammer Curls
		1 set of 21s
Sunday	Rest	Cardio on treadmill for 45 minutes

Week 5

Day of the Week		Exercises
Monday	Chest, Shoulders and Triceps	Barbell Bench Press
		Incline Bench Press
		20 Push-ups on Toes
		Standing Front Raises
		Bent-over Side Laterals
		Standing Push-Press with Barbell
		Triceps Extension
		Overhead Dumbbell
		Tricep kick-backs
Tuesday	Legs, Abs	Warm up legs by marching in place and doing side-to-sides for 5 minutes or by running outside for 10 minutes
		Plié squats
		Single legged squats
		Walking lunges with dumbbells
		Leg Presses (to 90 degrees)
		Side plank twists x 3
		Reverse crunches with an exercise ball x 3
		Hold plank on toes for 1 minute, rest 1 minute x 3
Wednesday	Rest	(Optional) Moms with babies: stroller walk for 45 minutes
		Moms with older kids: Cardio on treadmill or stationary bike for 45 minutes

Thursday	Back and Biceps	Deadlifts with Triple Rows (*high risk)
		Reverse grip Deadlift Rows (*high risk)
		Single Arm rows
		Bent-over Dumbbell Rows
		21s x 3
		Alternate Hammer Curls
		Switch to plate lifts and twist at the top
		Regular bicep curls to failure for last set
Friday	Cardio	Moms with babies: stroller walk for 45 minutes
		Moms with older kids: Cardio on treadmill or stationary bike for 45 minutes
Saturday	Chest, Shoulders and Triceps	Barbell Bench Press
		Incline Bench Press
		Pec Dec
		Standing Front Raises
		Standing Side Laterals
		Sitting Shoulder Press with Dumbbells
		Triceps Extension
		Overhead Dumbbell
		Tricep kick-backs
Sunday	Rest	25 Minutes Elliptical Trainer; 25 Minutes Treadmill Intervals

Week 6

Day of the Week		Exercises
Monday	Legs, Abs (Big muscle groups)	Standing Squats with Barbell
		Standing Squats with Ball on the Wall (go lower to 90 degrees)
		Reverse Lunges on Bench with Dumbbells (use 12s or 15s)
		Squats off Side of Bench with Lateral Leg Raises
		Jump Squats x 3
		Oblique Crunches x 3
		Slow Bicycles x 3
		Slow Straight Legged Sit-ups x 3
Tuesday	Back and Biceps	Wide-grip Lat Pulldowns (*high risk)
		Seated Cable or Dumbbell Rows
		Wide-grip Deadlift Rows (*high risk)
		Alternate Bicep Curls with Dumbbells
		Alternate Hammer Curls
		Band Bicep Curls
Wednesday	Rest	Moms with babies: stroller walk for 30 minutes
		Moms with older kids: Cardio on treadmill or stationary bike for 30 minutes
Thursday	Chest, Shoulders and Triceps	Cardio warm-up for 5 minutes
		20 Wide-grip Push-ups
		Barbell Chest Presses
		Incline Dumbbell Presses
		Standing Shoulder Presses (*high risk)
		Standing Lateral Raises
		Plié Squats with Front Raises
		Triceps Kick-backs
		Triceps Extensions
		Bench Dips to Failure x 1

Friday	Cardio	Moms with babies: stroller walk for 45 minutes
		Moms with older kids: Cardio on treadmill or stationary bike for 45 minutes
Saturday	Legs, Abs (Smaller muscle groups)	Stationary Lunges with Dumbbells
		Plié Squats; last set 16 pulses, then isometric hold for 15 sec.
		Lateral Lunges with Heavy Dumbbell
		Seated Ball Squeezes
		Band Side-to-Side Walks
		20 Bent Knee Crunches x 3
		20 In-and-Outs x 3
		20 Starfishes x 3
Sunday	Rest	Moms with babies: stroller walk for 45 minutes
		Moms with older kids: Cardio on treadmill or stationary bike for 45 minutes

Week 7

Day of the Week		Exercises
Monday	Back and Biceps, Abs	Hyperextensions (*high risk)
		Bent-Over Barbell Rows (*high risk)
		Seated Cable or Band Rows
		Preacher Curls
		Standing Dumbbell Curls
		Concentration Dumbbell Curls
		Bent-Knee Crunches x 3
		Reverse Crunches with Ball x 3
		Hold Planks x 3 (1 min. each)
Tuesday	Chest, Shoulders and Triceps	Barbell Bench Press
		Pec Dec / Rotators
		20 Wide Angle Push-ups x 3
		Seated Dumbbell Press
		Seated Dumbbell Side Laterals (arms bent)
		Plié Squats with Front Raises
		Lying Barbell Extension (narrow grip)
		Overhead Dumbbell Extension
		20 Triceps Push-ups x 3
Wednesday	Rest	Moms with babies: stroller walk for 45 minutes
		Moms with older kids: Cardio on treadmill or stationary bike for 45 minutes
Thursday	Legs, Abs	Barbell Squats (hip width)
		Reverse Lunges off Bench holding Dumbbell, knee lift
		Donkey Kicks
		Standing Calf Raises with Dumbbells (3 angles)
		20 Ab Crunches x 3
		20 Reverse Crunches x 3
		20 In and Outs x 3 with a dumbbell

Friday	Cardio	Sprint intervals on treadmill or outside, or turbo kickboxing
Saturday	Back and Biceps	Underhand Pull-downs (*high risk)
		Bent-over Dumbbell Rows
		Barbell Deadlifts (*high risk)
		Standing Dumbbell Curls
		Concentration Dumbbell Curls
		Standing Hammer Curls
		1 set of 21s
Sunday	Rest	Cardio on treadmill for 45 minutes

Week 8

Day of the Week		Exercises
Monday	Chest, Shoulders and Triceps	Dumbbell Bench Press
		Incline Dumbbell Bench Press
		Flat Flys
		Standing Push-Press with Barbell (*high risk)
		Seated Shoulder Presses with Dumbbells
		Standing Side Laterals
		Overhead Dumbbell
		20 Bench Dips x 3
		Triceps kick-backs
Tuesday	Legs, Abs	Warm up legs by marching in place and doing side-to-sides for 5 minutes or by running outside for 10 minutes
		Donkey Kicks
		Single legged squats
		Pulse Squats
		20 Jump Squats x 3
		Walking lunges with dumbbells
		Side plank twists x 3
		Reverse Crunches with an exercise ball x 3
		Hold plank on toes for 1 minute, rest 1 minute x 3
Wednesday	Rest	Moms with babies: stroller walk for 45 minutes
		Moms with older kids: Cardio on treadmill or stationary bike for 45 minutes

Thursday	Back and Biceps	Deadlifts with Triple Rows (*high risk)
		Incline Single Arm rows
		Bent-over Dumbbell Rows
		Push-up Rows w/ Dumbbells x 3
		21s x 3
		Alternate Hammer Curls
		Concentration Dumbbell Curls
		Regular bicep curls to failure for last set
Friday	Cardio	1 minute of jumping jacks
		1 minute rest
		Bench Side-to-Side Jumps
		1 minute rest
		10 Burpees with tuck jump
		20 minute intervals on the elliptical
Saturday	Chest, Shoulders and Triceps	20 Wide-grip Push-ups
		Pec Dec / Rotators
		Incline Dumbbell Flys
		Standing Front Raises
		Standing Shoulder Presses
		Standing Side Laterals
		20 Triceps Push-ups x 3
		Lying Barbell Extension (narrow grip)
		Overhead Triceps Extension
Sunday	Rest	25 Minutes Elliptical Trainer; 25 Minutes Treadmill Intervals

Week 9

Day of the Week		Exercises
Monday	Legs, Abs (Big muscle groups)	Standing Squats with Barbell
		Standing Squats with Ball on the Wall (go lower to 90 degrees)
		Single Leg Squats
		One Set of Walking Lunges to Failure (no added weight)
		Jump Squats x 3
		Oblique Crunches x 3
		Tabata Drill – bicycles, scissors, swimmers
Tuesday	Back and Biceps	Wide-grip Lat Pulldowns (*high risk)
		Seated Cable or Dumbbell Rows
		Wide-grip Deadlift Rows (*high risk)
		Alternate Bicep Curls with Dumbbells
		Alternate Hammer Curls
		Band Bicep Curls to Failure (one set)
Wednesday	Rest	Moms with babies: stroller walk for 45 minutes
		Moms with older kids: Cardio on treadmill or stationary bike for 45 minutes
Thursday	Chest, Shoulders and Triceps	Incline Dumbbell Presses
		Standing Shoulder Presses
		Standing Lateral Raises
		Plié Squats with Front Raises
		Triceps Kick-backs
		Triceps Extension
		20 Triceps Push-ups x 3
Friday	Cardio	Turbo kickboxing or interval training with plyos

Saturday	Legs, Abs (Smaller muscle groups)	Stationary Lunges with Dumbbells
		Plié Squats, then pulse, then hold
		Single Leg Squats
		Seated Ball Squeezes
		Band Side-to-Side Walks
		Bent Knee Crunches x 3
		Side-to-Side Dumbbell Crunches
		Reverse Crunches with the Ball
Sunday	Rest	Moms with babies: stroller walk for 45 minutes
		Moms with older kids: Cardio on treadmill or stationary bike for 45 minutes

Week 10

Day of the Week		Exercises
Monday	Back and Biceps, Abs	Hyperextensions (*high risk)
		Bent-Over Barbell Rows (*high risk)
		Seated Cable or Band Rows
		Preacher Curls
		Standing Dumbbell Curls
		Standing Hammer Curls
		Bent-Knee Crunches x 3
		Reverse Crunches with Ball x 3
		Hold Planks x 3 (1 min. each)
Tuesday	Chest, Shoulders and Triceps	Barbell Bench Press
		Pec Dec / Rotators
		20 Wide Angle Push-ups x 3
		Seated Dumbbell Press
		Bent-Over Dumbbell Side Laterals
		Plié Squats with Front Raises
		Lying Barbell Extension (narrow grip)
		Overhead Dumbbell Extension 20 Triceps Push-ups x 3
Wednesday	Rest	Moms with babies: stroller walk for 45 minutes
		Moms with older kids: Cardio on treadmill or stationary bike for 45 minutes / Walk with Baby for 45 Minutes
Thursday	Legs, Abs	Barbell Squats (hip width)
		Reverse Lunges off Bench holding Dumbbell, knee lift
		Leg Curls or Donkey Kicks
		Standing Calf Raises with Dumbbells (3 angles)
		20 Ab crunches x 3
		20 Reverse Crunches x 3
		20 In and Outs x 3 with a dumbbell

Friday	Cardio	Sprint intervals on treadmill or outside, or turbo kickboxing
Saturday	Back and Biceps	Wide-grip Deadlift Rows *(high risk)
		Barbell Deadlifts (*high risk)
		Bent-over Dumbbell Rows
		Standing Dumbbell Curls
		Concentration Dumbbell Curls
		Alternate Hammer Curls
		1 set of 21s
Sunday	Rest	Cardio on treadmill for 45 minutes

Week 11

Day of the Week		Exercises
Monday	Chest, Shoulders and Triceps	Barbell Bench Press
		Incline Dumbbell Bench Press
		Flat Flys
		Standing Push-Press with Barbell (*high risk)
		Seated Shoulder Presses with Dumbbells
		Standing Side Laterals
		Overhead Dumbbell
		Triceps Extension
		Triceps kick-backs
Tuesday	Legs, Abs	Warm up legs by marching in place and doing side-to-sides for 5 minutes or by running outside for 10 minutes
		Barbell Wide Squats
		Single legged squats
		Pulse Squats
		20 Jump Squats x 3
		Walking lunges with dumbbells
		Side plank twists x 3
		Reverse Crunches with an exercise ball x 3
		Hold plank on toes for 1 minute, rest 1 minute x 3
Wednesday	Rest	Moms with babies: stroller walk for 45 minutes
		Moms with older kids: Cardio on treadmill or stationary bike for 45 minutes

Thursday	Back and Biceps	Deadlifts with Triple Rows (*high risk)
		Single Arm rows
		Bent-over Dumbbell Rows
		Push-up Rows w/ Dumbbells x 3
		21s x 3
		Alternate Hammer Curls
		Concentration Dumbbell Curls
		Regular bicep curls to failure for last set
Friday	Cardio	1 minute of jumping jacks
		1 minute rest
		Bench Side-to-Side Jumps
		1 minute rest
		10 Burpees with tuck jump
		20 minute intervals on the elliptical
Saturday	Chest, Shoulders and Triceps	20 Wide-grip Push-ups
		Pec Dec / Rotators
		Flat Barbell Flys
		Standing Front Raises
		Standing Shoulder Presses
		Standing Barbell Presses
		20 Triceps Push-ups x 3
		Lying Barbell Extension (narrow grip) Overhead Triceps Extension
		1 Set of Kickbacks to Failure
Sunday	Rest	25 Minutes Elliptical Trainer; 25 Minutes Treadmill Intervals

Week 12

Day of the Week		Exercises
Monday	Legs, Abs (Big muscle groups)	Standing Squats with Barbell
		Standing Squats with Ball on the Wall (go lower to 90 degrees)
		Reverse Lunges on Bench with Dumbbells (use 12s or 15s)
		Squats off Side of Bench with Lateral Leg Raises
		Jump Squats x 3
		Oblique Crunches x 3
		Slow Bicycles x 3
		Slow Straight Legged Sit-ups x 3
Tuesday	Back and Biceps	Wide-grip Lat Pulldowns (*high risk)
		Seated Cable or Dumbbell Rows
		Wide-grip Deadlift Rows (*high risk)
		Alternate Bicep Curls with Dumbbells
		Alternate Hammer Curls
		Band Bicep Curls
		Standing Dumbbell Curls to Failure (last set)
Wednesday	Rest	Moms with babies: stroller walk for 45 minutes
		Moms with older kids: Cardio on treadmill or stationary bike for 45 minutes
Thursday	Chest, Shoulders and Triceps	Cardio warm-up for 5 minutes
		20 Wide-grip Push-ups
		Barbell Chest Presses
		Incline Dumbbell Presses
		Standing Dumbbell Shoulder Presses
		Pec Dec
		Plié Squats with Front Raises
		Overhead Dumbbell
		Triceps Extensions
		Bench Dips to Failure x 1

Friday	Cardio	Moms with babies: stroller walk for 45 minutes
		Moms with older kids: Cardio on treadmill or stationary bike for 45 minutes
Saturday	Legs, Abs (Smaller muscle groups)	Stationary Lunges with Dumbbells
		Plié Squats; last set 16 pulses, then isometric hold for 15 sec.
		Single Leg Squats
		Donkey Kicks
		Band Side-to-Side Walks
		20 Bent Knee Crunches x 3
		20 In-and-Outs x 3
		20 Starfishes x 3
Sunday	Rest	Moms with babies: stroller walk for 45 minutes
		Moms with older kids: Cardio on treadmill or stationary bike for 45 minutes

LET'S CONNECT

As my Thank You to you for buying this book, I want to give you an awesome free bonus. It's a fully interactive and printable cookbook, featuring some great, yummy Fit Mom Recipes over the course of 30 days. This will help to take the stress out of planning healthy meals for you and your family.

Go to link:
FitMomSecrets.com/FreeFitMomCookbook

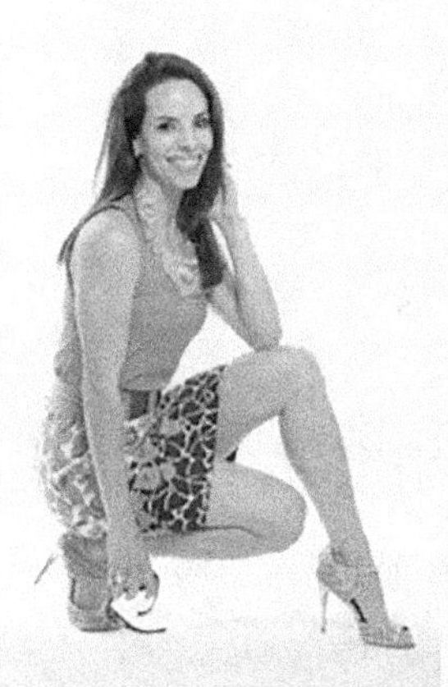

Please connect with me on my public Facebook page at *Facebook.com/SecretsOfTheSuperMom*. This is where I often post some of my best fitness tips, live workout videos, and demo healthy recipes. It's also a great place to connect with other moms who have similar goals as you.

I hope reading this book has been a worthwhile investment of your time. It's the culmination of my lifelong interest in health and fitness and helping other moms create healthy homes. If you've enjoyed it and will apply some of the lessons I teach here, I'd greatly appreciate it if you would write a review on Amazon. The more moms who can get a copy of **Fit Mom Secrets**, the more healthy families we'll have, and that includes our children who deserve the absolute best from all of us.

Official Secrets of the Super Mom Facbook Fanpage

http://www.facbook.com/SecretsOfTheSuperMom

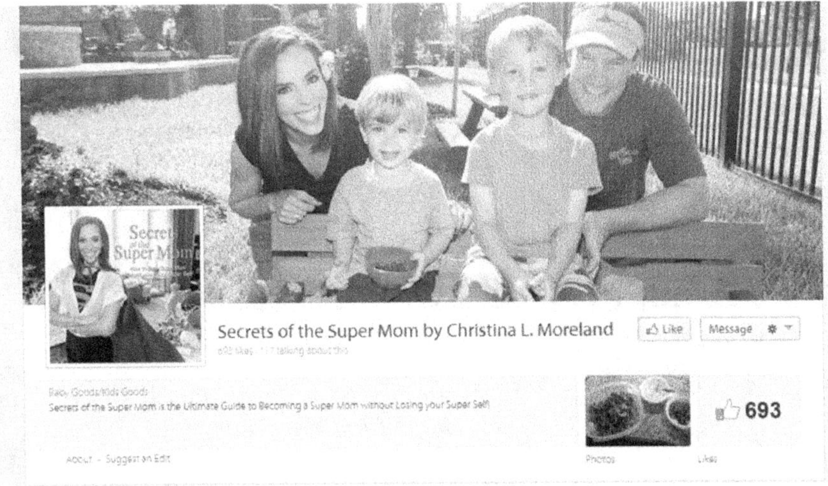

Other Books by Christina L. Moreland

Secrets of the Super Moms, Part 1: How To Be a Super Mom Without Losing Your Super Self in the First Two Years

Secrets of the Super Moms, Part 2: Finances, Fitness, Fashion and More!

For more information, visit *www.SecretsOfTheSuperMoms.com*